Disaster Evaluation Research

T0177505

Disaster Evaluation Research
A Field Guide

Edmund M. Ricci
Ernesto A. Pretto, Jr.
Knut Ole Sundnes

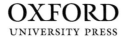

OXFORD
UNIVERSITY PRESS

OXFORD
UNIVERSITY PRESS

Great Clarendon Street, Oxford, OX2 6DP,
United Kingdom

Oxford University Press is a department of the University of Oxford.
It furthers the University's objective of excellence in research, scholarship,
and education by publishing worldwide. Oxford is a registered trade mark of
Oxford University Press in the UK and in certain other countries

First Edition published in 2019

Impression: 1

Published in the United States of America by Oxford University Press
198 Madison Avenue, New York, NY 10016, United States of America

British Library Cataloguing in Publication Data

Data available

Library of Congress Control Number: 2019937521

ISBN 978-0-19-879686-2

Printed and bound by
CPI Group (UK) Ltd, Croydon, CR0 4YY

Preface

Following every major disaster—whether a devastating flood, a powerful earthquake, a massive hurricane, or a voracious wildfire—many stories are told. Some are deeply personal accounts by survivors of the frightening experience of living through the disaster, and many of these quickly find their way into the public domain. In addition, there are always descriptions prepared by journalists, usually broader in scope than those prepared by survivors, that document the wider human toll of the disaster upon the affected population. Often, journalists are able to identify rescue attempts that have not worked as well as hoped, resulting in unnecessary injury and loss of life; or they may describe dramatic and emotionally moving rescues.

Other narratives may be prepared by those trained in any one of several scientific disciplines. Social scientists, for example, may describe the immediate and long-term suffering of those who lived within the disaster zone, calculating and describing the human toll, or the impact upon community infrastructure, cohesion, and resilience. Scientists, trained in the methods of public health research, might focus their efforts upon the victims, describing in quantitative terms the loss of life and the disability, both mental and physical, that followed the horrific conditions associated with the disaster event. Engineers trained in structural engineering science may seek to understand the processes of building collapse, with analysis of the factors resulting in damage to individuals trapped or pinned under rubble.

One highly important narrative, however, has seldom been fully told. Public health professionals who are trained and experienced in using the methods of 'evaluation science' have only rarely been able to apply the methods and concepts of their special area of expertise to scientifically assess the medical and public health response to a disaster. Without doubt disasters present a particularly difficult arena for the application of evaluation science, and, to add to the difficulty, there is little methodological guidance in the evaluation science literature about how to do so. Further, in those rare occasions when comprehensive disaster evaluation studies have been conducted, they have had little impact upon ongoing and future disaster preparedness and response efforts.

Therefore, the ultimate hope, and great challenge, undertaken by the authors of this volume is to improve disaster preparedness and response efforts globally by providing a standardized way to conduct rigorous and comprehensive scientific evaluation studies of the medical and public health response. We maintain our deeply held belief that the widespread application of the lessons learned from studies that are fully grounded in 'evaluation science' will result in more effective preparedness and response which, in turn, will bring about a universally desired reduction in disaster related death, disability, and suffering.

Inspiration and Vision

This volume has been inspired by the untiring efforts of Peter Safar, MD, in his relentless life-quest to work toward the humanitarian goal that, in his words, 'no one shall die before their time'. His pioneering and ground-breaking work in mouth-to-mouth resuscitation (rescue breathing) in the 1950s was the impetus for the subsequent development of many life-saving innovations such as cardiopulmonary resuscitation (CPR), pre-hospital emergency care systems, mobile intensive care ambulances, and the medical specialties of Emergency and Critical Care Medicine, which ultimately led him into a deep and longstanding interest in preventing loss of life following large-scale disasters.

Safar's early case studies of the causes of morbidity and mortality following earthquakes in Peru (1970) and Italy (1980) convinced him that more lives could be saved following such disasters if modern concepts and procedures of emergency and critical care medicine could be applied in a more routine and systematic fashion. The great Armenian earthquake of 1988, which resulted in more than 75,000 casualties with an inverse ratio of killed to injured of 3:1, further motivated Dr. Safar to continue his quest to learn more about the causes of disaster-related morbidity and mortality.

Until recently, in many corners of the world, the negative impact of disasters was accepted as fate. In other words, the resulting human and economic losses were considered irreducible. The attitude toward disaster was viewed as 'divine punishment' or considered to be the invisible hand of God, as mirrored in the term 'Acts of God'. This thinking reflected an earlier focus on natural disasters. However, during the period 1996–2015, 1.35 million people were killed in more than 7,000 natural disasters throughout our planet. As public health and medical professionals began to take notice of morbidity and mortality data that revealed the immense size and frequency of the impact on the health of human populations, it was natural that they should ask: Can we do better with saving lives and minimizing death and injury, and preventing public health-related calamity in major disasters?

Thus, the specialties of Emergency and Critical Care Medicine and Public Health Preparedness and Response converged to establish the field of Disaster Medicine. Disaster Medicine is a relatively new field within the spectrum of the health/public health professions, comprising many disciplines that deal with the medical and public health consequences of disasters. As a result, many concepts, terminology, curricula for educational and training programs, and procedures have not yet been standardized or broadly agreed with; nor are practices firmly rooted in science.

Also, as of this writing there continue to be few comprehensive training programs in Disaster Medicine and Disaster Management. In the United States the Association of Schools of Public Health published the first disaster preparedness curriculum for schools of public health in 2001 (Landesman, 2001). Currently several schools of Public Health offer courses in disaster preparedness and response, and some of these offer full certificate programs. The "European Masters in Disaster Medicine," which draws students globally, is offered by the faculty of medicine and pharmacy at Vrije Universiteit, Brussel Laarbeeklaan, Belgium and the Universitá del Piemonte Orientale, Amadeo Avagadro, Novara, Italy.

In 1994, the Norwegian Association for Disaster Medicine, and the Nordic Society for Disaster Medicine created an independent task force with international membership drawn from NATO and the World Association for Disaster and Emergency Medicine, among others. This group evolved into the 'Task Force on Quality Control of Disaster Management' (TFQCDM) whose members continue to work to improve the quality of disaster preparedness and response globally. This Field Manual is an extension of their interest in applying scientific evaluation concepts and methods in order to advance the goal of decreasing death and injury resulting from disasters.

What Do We Hope to Accomplish With This Book?

It is our firm belief that the framework for evaluation developed by specialists in scientific evaluation, based upon a 'program theory' as portrayed in a logic model, offers the most appropriate and comprehensive structure for disaster evaluation studies. This conceptual framework is now widely adapted and used by public health organizations internationally as a basis for the evaluation of medical, public health, and community-based interventions. We believe that many more disaster-related deaths and injuries can be prevented if the concepts and methods of 'scientific evaluation' are applied to the disaster situation.

The approach we describe in this Field Manual has not been widely used in its entirety in disaster evaluation studies. In part this is because there does not yet exist a book that describes the application of a comprehensive approach, drawing upon scientific evaluation concepts and methods, to assess the medical and public health response to a multi-casualty disaster.

We take this opportunity, then, to describe in Part 1 of this book the basic concepts and scientific framework used by program evaluation scientists. In doing so we have drawn upon the several evaluation scientists who have contributed greatly to the specialty of evaluation.

We then, in Part 2, follow our description of scientific program evaluation, with an illustration of how scientific evaluation methods and concepts may be applied to a disaster event in order to assess the process (intervention) and effectiveness (outcomes) of the medical and public health response to these horrific events.

We hope what will ultimately follow the widespread application of comprehensive scientific evaluation methods is a global improvement in the medical and public health response to disasters. However, we are not so naïve as to believe that disaster preparedness and response will change as a direct result of the availability of scientifically grounded assessments. Change requires a double-pronged commitment—leaders from the ranks both of politics and of public health must carefully consider, adopt, and fund policy positions and programs based upon the findings and recommendations that emerge from scientific evaluation studies.

We have struggled for a long time to determine how best to apply evaluation science in disaster settings because disasters present an unusually difficult situation in which to attempt rigorous scientific evaluation. However, we continue to be guided and motivated by the spirit and momentum of Dr. Safar's great humanitarian journey to assure that 'no one shall die before their time'.

Reference

Landesman, L.Y., ed. (2001). *Public Health Response to Disasters: A Curriculum for the New Millennium.* Washington, DC: Association of Schools of Public Health.

Resources with this book

This book includes useful tools for carrying out evaluations including; evaluation questions, indicators and data sources, resources, and questionnaires used in past evaluation studies. Copies of these documents are available as downloadable interactive PDFs at www.oxfordmedicine.com/disaster

Acknowledgements

The work described in this book has been inspired by the efforts of the Task Force on Quality Control on Disaster Management (TFQCDM), a group of international experts who have participated in a series of consensus conferences held between 1995 and 2016 at the Utstein Abby, Stavanger 14, Norway at the Nordic School of Public Health, Gothenburg, Sweden. These workshops were sponsored by the Nordic International Rescue Foundation, the Laerdal Foundation for Acute Medicine, the Norwegian Armed Forces Medical Services, the Swedish National Board on Health and Welfare, the Swedish International Developing Agency (SIDA), and the Nordic Council.

This book is an elaboration of the essential elements of an evaluative field methodology, derived from evaluation science, to improve the scientific rigor of emergency public health and disaster medicine research as defined by the Utstein Style for guidelines. The Utstein Style label derives from a series of consensus conferences on disaster planning, preparedness, and evaluation, held at the Utstein Abbey, located on the Island of Mosteroy, Rogaland County, near the city of Stavanger, Norway. It was in this place that researchers from around the world, under the auspices of the European Society of Cardiology, met to develop guidelines for the uniform reporting of data from out-of-hospital cardiac arrest. These Utstein cardiac arrest guidelines and templates have significantly advanced the science of cardiac arrest.

The TFQCDM has intended to do for Disaster Medicine what others have done for cardiac arrest, namely to provide a solid scientific foundation upon which to improve the practice. The authors of this book are members of the TFQCDM while Dr. Knut Ole Sundnes continues to serve as Chairman of the group.

This book is also loosely based on a field research survey methodology, first applied by a group of multidisciplinary experts at the University of Pittsburgh after the 1988 Armenia earthquake, and later refined and applied after earthquakes in Costa Rica and Turkey. This assembly of academics and professional emergency medical practitioners organized themselves as the 'Disaster Reanimatology Study Group' of the International Resuscitation Research Center then directed by Dr. Peter Safar. Edmund Ricci and Ernesto A. Pretto Jr. were founding members of this group.

We acknowledge the following members of the TFQCDM who have supported and contributed to the present iteration of the disaster evaluation field methodology described in this book.

Dag Hjelle, MD, Brigadier General and Director Norwegian Armed Forces Joint Medical Services

Yasufumi Asai, MD, Emeritus Professor, Sapporo Medical University, Japan Special advisor of Japan Disaster Relief (JICA) and Editor in Chief of Journal of Japan Association of Disaster

Robert Balazs, MD, Lt. Col. Technical Officer (Medical) NATO Operational Logistics Planning and Support Programme Office

Per Morten Boelstad, Lt. Col. Safety Inspector (Infantry) Norwegian Armed Forces joint medical services/risk, safety, preparedness, and vulnerability

Felipe Cruz Vega, MD, Mexican Institute of Social Security, Special Health Projects Division

David Siddarth, Senior Research Officer, School of Habitat Studies, Tata Institute of Social Sciences (TISS), Mumbai, India

Michel Debacker, MD, Professor and Director, Research Group on Emergency and Disaster Medicine, Faculty of Medicine and Pharmacy, Vrije Universiteit, Brussel Laarbeeklaan, Belgium

Hon. Emmanuel de Guzman, Philippine Climate Change Commissioner, Philippine Climate Change Commission, San Miguel, Manila, Philippines

S. William A. Gunn, MD, Former Director, Emergency Humanitarian Operations, WHO, Geneva, and member Academic Council of the United Nations System

Christian Haggenmiller, MD, Lecturer and Colonel, Bundeswehr Command and Staff College, formerly with the NATO Joint Analysis and Lessons Learned Center

Leo Klein, MD, PhD, Associate Professor and Brigadier General, Former Surgeon General of the Czech Armed Forces, Dept. of Military Surgery, Faculty of Military Health Sciences, University Hospital Hradec Králové, Czech Republic, Dept. of Surgery, Division of Plastic Reconstructive Surgery and Burns Treatment

Istvan Kopcso MD, PhD, Brigadier General, Medical Advisor Supreme Headquarters, Allied Powers Europe Belgium

Isidore K. Kouadio, MD, PhD, FETP, DMHA Regional Polio Certification Officer, Global Polio Eradication Initiative

Omar Juma Khatib, MD,WHO Regional Office for Africa, Brazzaville, Republic of Congo

Håkon Lund, MD, Lt. Col., Senior Staff Officer, Norwegian Armed Forces Medical Services

Ove Njå, PhD, Professor, University of Stavanger

Nobhojit Roy, MB, Professor and Head of Surgical Services and Scientist 'G' BARC Hospital, HBNI University, Mumbai, India

Sidika Tekeli, MD, Assistant Professor, Head of Department Hacettepe, University Institute of Public Health, Department of Health Management in Disasters, Turkey

Andreas Ziegler, MD MSc EMDM MBA, Vienna Municipal Ambulance Service

Jeffrey Arnold, MD, Chief Medical Officer, Santa Clara Valley Health and Hospital System, Santa Clara County, California, USA

Johan Calltorp, MD, PhD, Professor, Nordic School of Public Health and Joenkoeping Academy (deceased)

While Dr. Peter Safar provided the vision and inspiration for this book, much of our thinking and conceptual formulation has been based upon the intellectual and ground-breaking efforts of two highly influential evaluation scientists, namely Drs. Edward Suchman and Michael Q. Patton. Our deep indebtedness to their remarkable efforts to create and improve evaluation science will be clear to those who make their way through this Field Manual.

We are extremely grateful to Dr. Todd Bear, Co-Director of the Evaluation Institute for Public Health, Graduate School of Public Health, University of Pittsburgh. Dr. Bear provided excellent suggestions for Chapters 9 (Sampling) and 12 (Data Analysis and Final Report) which we have adopted, and he helped with the conceptualization of Part 2 of this book. He has thereby been an important intellectual guide and supporter for this effort. Tom McClure reviewed Part 1 and provided numerous suggestions that improved the clarity of the text.

Alisa Vinje assisted with the preparation of the entire manuscript by carrying out extensive editorial and word processing tasks, with a large dose of patience, as we continuously revised the content and wording. Without her energy and skilled technical support, it is hard to imagine that this book would have yet taken final form. Dr. Nora Bridges provided inestimable assistance in the preparation of the final manuscript. Her editorial and substantive contributions were essential to the completion of this book.

Carson Hawk, Celeste Petruzzi, Chantel Durant, Jesse Evans, Leigh Bukowski, and Danielle Ferry provided assistance in the preparation of this manuscript while also adding large amounts of encouragement. We are especially grateful for their contributions which cannot be adequately described and acknowledged.

Edmund Ricci
Ernesto A. Pretto, Jr.
Knut Ole Sundnes

Contents

Abbreviations

AEA	American Evaluation Association		ICS	incident command system
ATLS	advanced trauma life support		ICU	intensive care unit
BSF	basic societal support functions		IMS	incident management system
CCP	casualty collection points		IRB	Institutional Review Board
CDC	Centers for Disease Control and Prevention		JCAHO	Joint Committee for Accreditation of Healthcare Organizations
CIOMS	Council for International Organizations of Medical Sciences		NATO	North Atlantic Treaty Organization
CRED	Center for Research on the Epidemiology of Disasters		NGO	non-governmental organization
DHHS	Department of Health and Human Services		PAHO	Pan American Health Organization
ESF	emergency support functions		SMART	(Objectives) specific, measurable, attainable, results oriented, within a timeframe
EMS	emergency medical services			
ERT	evaluation research team		TFQCDM	Task force on quality control of disaster management
GDP	gross domestic product			

Part 1

A Comprehensive Framework for Disaster Evaluation

In Part 1 of this field manual, we place this book within the historical context of disaster research (Chapter 1) and then, in Chapters 2 and 3, a general framework for scientific evaluation is described. In Chapter 4 the components of a comprehensive medical and public health response system are identified.

The concepts and frameworks described in Part 1 provide the background for Part 2, in which an 'Eight-Step Model' for disaster evaluation is presented and discussed, step by step, as guidance to those who will follow our approach in the future.

This Field Manual concludes with a discussion of ethical issues which should be addressed by those doing disaster evaluation studies (Chapter 13) and a look to the future of disaster evaluation research in Chapter 14 (Epilogue).

Chapter 1

A Brief History of Disaster Evaluation Studies

Keypoints

The scientific study of disasters has a long history, albeit limited in scope and structure. The first studies tended to focus on the societal and human impact of these horrific events and to report numbers of casualties. Later studies examined more deeply the impact and stresses disasters have placed upon the individuals and communities affected and upon the emergency public health and medical care systems in the affected geographic areas. The methodological challenges to conducting these studies have been great in that disasters are typically unexpected, and there is little time for recording and collecting data concurrently. However, a methodology for collecting data descriptive of the medical and public health response to disasters is evolving through much trial and error. This chapter is not intended to be a comprehensive review of disaster evaluation research and evaluation. It is, rather, a portrait of some highlights in the complex and difficult pathway traversed by those who have attempted to study disasters while using the methods of science.

Introduction

The International Task Force on Quality Control of Disaster Management, drawing upon the work of others, have defined a disaster as:

> a serious disruption of the functioning of society causing wide spread human, material, economic or environmental losses which exceed the ability of the affected society to cope using only its own resources.

(Sundnes, 2014)

While the international community has made progress in defining the components of a comprehensive public health and medical response system, the terminology employed to describe disaster response functions has not been fully agreed upon. We have decided to use definitions provided by the Task Force on Quality Control of Disaster Management (TFQCDM) because they stem from the efforts of an international group of disaster medicine and public health professionals whose collective experience is vast.

These definitions focus upon two characteristics of a societal/community disaster: (1) it is an event that overwhelms the society/community affected by the event; and (2) outside assistance is required in order to cope with the destruction which occurs. A third characteristic that follows is that disasters have an impact upon the health and safety of the affected population, as well as societal cohesion and infrastructure, thereby pushing individual and community resilience capacity to the limit and beyond.

Disasters may be caused by naturally occurring events or by human activity. They may vary in duration from "short" (earthquake, tsunami, volcanic eruption, structural failure, and avalanche) to long term (floods, disease epidemics, drought, famine, armed conflict).

Disaster preparedness is 'the aggregate of all measures and policies taken by humans before the event occurs (in order to) reduce the damage that otherwise would have been caused by the event' (Sundnes and Birnbaum 2003).

Disaster response is typically defined as 'the aggregate of all measures taken to cope with the damage sustained' (Sundnes and Birnbaum 2003). In this book, however, we focus primarily on the medical and public health components of the total disaster response.

Historical Highlights

Historically, disasters have not been easily accessible for study by scientific researchers. However, the landmark doctoral dissertation of Dr. Samuel Henry Prince on the Halifax explosion in 1917, which caused 1,963 deaths and injured 9,000 others (comprising 20% of the population), was among the first attempts to examine a disaster from a scholarly perspective (Prince 1920). Prince was a doctoral student in sociology at that time. His focus, however, was to address the social aspects of the disaster and in so doing he developed a theory of collective behavior during disaster situations. T. Joseph Scanlon in a 1988 article described Prince's pioneering work and his role as an originator of disaster research.

> Prince dealt with many of the things which are now regarded as critical to collective behavior. He alluded to disaster subculture, he discussed the possibility of internal and external strains, he referred to the structure of society.

> (Scanlon, 1988)

Obviously inspired by Prince, T. Joseph Scanlon (1988) assessed the response to mass death after the 1917 Halifax explosion. Scanlon, writing from the perspective of his position as Director, Emergency Communications Research Unit, Canada, focused upon how victims' bodies are handled following disasters in which there are large numbers of rapidly occurring deaths, a highly important public health concern.

In the time span from 1920 to 1980 a small number of social scientists did study disasters from their separate and different disciplinary platforms. Public health and medical response issues were not a primary focus. Also, since the academic establishment that was involved in medical research promoted the randomized controlled trial as the 'gold standard' for reproducible clinical research, a study of the health and medical response to the challenges posed by disasters tended to be seen as insurmountable because controlled trials are not possible to implement under disaster conditions. Consequently, disaster papers and publications continued to be anecdotal, not peer reviewed and mostly only published in the 'grey literature'; however, slowly this changed.

Beginning in the 1980s, health-focused disaster research methodologies were enriched by the introduction of qualitative data collection methods as used routinely in the social sciences. It had become apparent that there was a need for more organized, systematic research specifically designed to assess the timeliness and adequacy of life-saving efforts provided by professional and non-professional emergency medical response teams in disaster conditions. Techniques commonly used in the social sciences began to be incorporated into disaster medicine and public health research. A wider variety of these methods is now available, which has led to improved data collection, quality, and interpretation. As a result, the scientific base of disaster evaluation is evolving from an anecdotal body of knowledge, to a more systematically obtained and analyzed body of information.

However, today disaster research, from a medical and public health perspective, still has largely had minimal impact upon disaster preparedness and response, not any longer because it is ignored, but due to the failure to identify and apply a comprehensive evaluation research framework and uniform data collection methods that are capable of capturing the huge web of complexity associated with disasters. Medical and public health journals which focus on somatic challenges in disasters are also few compared to journals addressing social and individual victim issues. Of the top journals globally that had included articles related to health issues in disasters between 1977 and 2009, only two of 16 had disasters as their prime focus. The others only occasionally included articles about disasters (Sundnes, 2014).

As with most fields of scientific inquiry, the scientific study of disasters has several roots. One of the longest and deepest of these roots can be found in the work of Enrico Quarantelli, Russell Dynes, and their associates in the Disaster Research Center. Founded in 1963, the group is now based at the University of Delaware. This group of social scientists has had a continuous record of scientific exploration and conceptual definition of human-generated and natural disasters. While their main focus has been on the societal, organizational, and human response, and the resulting consequences of disasters, in so doing they have defined the way we conceptualize the widespread impact of disasters upon community life during and following these major human tragedies. They also have produced a wealth of case study reports that are of great value to this effort (Quarantelli, 2002).

A focus upon the assessment of the medical and public health response to large-scale disasters began with the accumulation of what were essentially journalistic case studies. These were typically the efforts of interested eyewitnesses or single investigators, at times physicians, who prepared descriptive accounts of the events that occurred during and in the short-term after the disaster event. These reports were extremely valuable in that they provided a 'broad brush' look into the impact of the disaster as experienced by victims, uninjured community residents, professionals, and members of various governmental and non-governmental organizations that participated in the disaster response.

The tragic earthquake which struck three large cities in Soviet Armenia in 1988, resulting in more than 75,000 casualties, further motivated medical and public health professionals including Peter Safar and colleagues of the University of Pittsburgh, and Eric Noji, then of the US Centers for Disease Control, with colleagues at Johns Hopkins University (H. Armenian) and in Armenia (O. Oganessian), to continue the quest to learn more about the causes of disaster-related morbidity and mortality (Safar 1985; Noji et al, 1990).

Two of the authors of this volume (Ricci and Pretto) were challenged by Dr. Safar to design and carry out a large-scale scientific investigation of the Armenian earthquake. We initially responded to Dr. Safar's request with considerable trepidation because the methodological and logistical issues involved in such a study were formidable. Nevertheless Dr. Safar's enthusiasm for the project ultimately overcame our concerns. The resulting study ultimately involved a multidisciplinary (evaluation science, medicine, public health, engineering, and social science) and international team of investigators (United States and Soviet Union/Armenia).

As anticipated, implementing an evaluation study for the first time in a large-scale disaster was extremely challenging and the study was only partially successful. However, much was learned about the methodological and practical issues involved in doing disaster-related evaluation studies, including an effort to apply statistical sampling methods to the selection of respondents and victims of a disaster (Ricci et al., 1991). Following this initial attempt to apply scientific evaluation methods to assess the medical and public health response to the Armenian earthquake, we refined the overall approach and then conducted field survey studies after earthquakes in Costa Rica, Turkey, the United States (California), and Japan, each time learning more about how to apply a mixed-method approach towards the goal of improving disaster planning and response.

In the revised approach, in addition to open-ended interviews we conducted structured interviews using bilingual user-specified multiple-choice questions intended for four critical target groups who were intimately involved in the response effort: health care professionals, lay injured and uninjured survivors, disaster coordinators/managers, and search and rescue personnel. The refinements to the study design also included collection and careful review of available medical records and/or autopsy reports, and other relevant 'official' situation and after-action reports, as well as journalistic accounts. Also, because we were primarily concerned with determining deaths that could have been prevented (i.e., Safar's resuscitation potential) questionnaires were constructed with a logical progression of multiple-choice user-specified questions designed to elicit undocumented information with as much detail as possible from target individuals who witnessed or were involved in the care of victims who died 'slowly' in the out-of-hospital setting. Specific questions were on the location, timing of death, type of injuries, first aid employed, and mode of transport, if applicable (see appendix: victim-specific questionnaire/verbal autopsy). The responses from these questions were labeled and entered into Centers for Disease Control and Prevention Epi-info software. We then compiled all the information collected from medical records, agency and official records, journalistic accounts, and interviews with target groups to reconstruct events and to infer numbers and potential causes and circumstances of preventable deaths (Pretto et al., 1992, 1994; Angus et al., 1997; Aoki et al., 2004).

The approach used by the University of Pittsburgh team in disaster studies involved a combination of evaluation and epidemiological methods now referred to as a 'mixed-methods' scientific approach applied within an evaluation framework.

Also, using epidemiological methods exclusively, Dr. C. De Ville De Goyet with the Pan American Health Organization (PAHO), Drs. R. I. Glass and E. K. Noji, and colleagues based in the US Public Health Service, Centers for Disease Control and Prevention, among others, have documented the injury toll of large-scale disasters. In Europe, Dr. Michel Lechat founded the Center for Research on the Epidemiology of Disasters (CRED) in 1971. Based in the University of Louvain School Of Public Health in Brussels, Belgium, the Center houses a large database of disaster-related epidemiological studies.

Thus, we have seen a progression of the study of the medical and public aspects of disaster planning and response, from journalistic reporting to more scientific approaches, the newest of which blend methods, techniques, and disciplines found in the social and behavioral sciences, epidemiology, statistics, evaluation science, and medical research into a truly comprehensive evaluation approach such as described in this volume. These studies are complementing the large number of excellent social science-based studies which focus upon the human and societal impact of disasters including factors underlying community resilience to these destructive events.

We have also welcomed the design and implementation of engineering studies whose aim has been to improve the disaster resistance of community infrastructure, e.g. buildings, roads, dams, power supply water, and bridges. The results of disaster engineering research are leading to improvements in the built environment and they are leading to the prevention of and significant reductions in morbidity and mortality associated with disasters. Obviously, disaster-resistant infrastructure design results in more opportunities to save lives.

Summary

In this chapter we have touched upon only a few of the important episodes in the development of disaster evaluation methods and studies. Historically, disaster research has followed several paths. Social science-oriented studies have contributed much to our understanding of the societal and human impact of disasters. Engineering research has been contributing greatly to making the built environment more resilient. Public health, engineering, and medical research, all only relatively recently applied to disasters, can be expected in the future to lead to significantly improved preparedness and response with a resulting reduction in disaster-related morbidity and mortality. As time progresses all of the efforts will hopefully be made to act in concert in a global effort to reach the overarching goal of saving more lives during and after a disaster strikes.

References

Angus, D., Pretto, E., Abrams, J.I., et al. (1997). Epidemiologic Assessment of Building Collapse Pattern, Mortality, and Medical Response After the 1992 Earthquake in Erzincan, Turkey. *Prehospital and Disaster Medicine.* **12** (3), pp. 222–231.

Aoki N, Nishimura A., Pretto E.A., et al. (2004). Survival and Cost Analysis of Fatalities after the Kobe Earthquake in Japan. *Prehospital Emergency Care.* **8** (2), pp. 217–222.

Noji, E., Kelen, G. Armenian, H., et al. (1990). The 1988 Earthquake in Soviet Armenia: A Case Study. *Annals of Emergency Medicine.* **19** (8), pp. 891–897.

Pretto, E., Ricci, E., Safar, P., et al. (1992). Disaster Reanimatology Potentials: A Structured Interview Study in Armenia III: Results, Conclusions, and Recommendations. *Prehospital and Disaster Medicine.* **7** (4), pp. 327–338.

Pretto, E. A., Angus, D.C., Abrams, J. J., et al. (1994). An Analysis of Prehospital Mortality in An Earthquake. *Prehospital and Disaster Medicine.* **9** (2), pp 107–117.

Prince, S. (1920). *Catastrophe and Social Change.* New York: Columbia University. (Doctoral Dissertation).

Quarantelli, E.L. (2002). The disaster research center field studies of organized behavior in the crisis time period of disasters. In: **Stallings, R.A.**, ed., *Methods of Disaster Research.* Philadelphia, PA: XLibris, pp. 94–126.

Ricci, E., Pretto, E.A., Safar, P., et al. (1991). Disaster Reanimatology Potentials: A Structured Interview Study in Armenia II: A Method for Assessment of the Medical Response to Major Disasters. *Prehospital and Disaster Medicine.* **6** (2): pp. 159-166.

Safar, P. (1985). Resuscitation potentials in mass disasters. In: **Manni, C.**, **Magalini, S.I.**, eds., *Emergency and Disaster Medicine.* Berlin: Springer.

Scanlon, J. (1988). Disaster's Little-Known Pioneer: Canada's Samuel Henry Prince. *International Journal of Mass Emergencies and Disasters.* **6** (3), pp. 213–232.

Sundnes, K.O. and Birnbaum, M.L. (2003). Health Disaster Management: Guidelines for Evaluation and Research in the Utstein Style. *Prehospital and Disaster Medicine.* **17** (3), p. 44.

Sundnes, K.O., ed. (2014). Health Disaster Management: Guidelines for Evaluation and Research in the "Utstein Style". Structural Framework, Operational Framework and Preparedness. *Scandinavian Journal of Public Health.* **42** (14), p. 15.

Further reading

Rodriguez, H., Quarantelli, E.L., and Dynes, R.R. (2007). *Handbook of Disaster Research.* New York, NY: Springer.

Noji, E. Armenian, H., Oganessian, A. (1993). Issues of rescue and medical care following the 1988 Armenian earthquake. *International Journal of Epidemiology.* **22** (6), pp. 1070–1076.

Chapter 2

A General Framework for Evaluation

Keypoints

Evaluation science emerged in the 1960s as a conceptual framework and methodology for using scientific methods to assess the structure, operation, costs, and outcomes of public health and other social programs. Evaluation is both a scientific specialty, which follows the rules of science, and a profession that operates within a framework of quality and ethical standards. The great challenge for evaluation is not only to motivate organizations to more effectively and consistently conduct scientific evaluation studies but also to use what has been learned through such studies to redesign programs based upon evaluation findings. The ultimate purpose of scientific evaluation is to improve human health and well-being through the application of evaluation findings to the design and implementation of public health and all other human service programs.

Evaluation matters. Too often it has been an afterthought in WHO planning, seen as an optional luxury. This must now change, so that the role of evaluation is seen as an opportunity for organizational and individual learning, to improve performance and accountability for results and build our capacity for understanding why some programs and initiatives work, and why others do not. We should not be complacent. Consistent and high quality evaluation of our work is essential.
(Margaret Chan, WHO, 2013)

Introduction

We begin our description of a general framework for evaluation by differentiating among various types of research. Although no classification of research uses mutually exclusive categories, we find useful a classification offered by a World Health Organization–based team. They suggest the following scheme:

Types of research:

- **Basic science research**: research that is laboratory-based, such as testing of human biological materials. An example might be investigation of a genetic variant that confers vulnerability to an agent that is causing an epidemic.

- **Clinical research**: research in which participants (individuals or groups) are prospectively assigned to a health intervention, from drugs and biological products to devices and preventive programs. An example of clinical research would be a clinical trial of therapy for disaster survivors.

- **Health services and health systems research**: research concerned mainly with the administrative and social aspects of health and health care, including financial aspects. An example of a health services research project would be an investigation of the impact of dealing with an epidemic on hospital performance.

- **Population-based research**: research on individuals in a wider context, which includes epidemiological surveillance and cohort studies and investigations of the impact of social determinants of health. An example of population-based research would be a study of the health outcomes of children who lived through a disaster.

- **Policy and advocacy research**: research on how evidence can best be transformed into practice and used to improve public health. A question for this type of research might be: 'Can social media be used to improve disaster preparedness?'

(World Health Organization, 2015)

An evaluation study of the medical and public health response to disasters would usually be considered a type of health services or health systems research that can be used to improve both policy choices and the preparation and response to disasters. However, methods and concepts used in other types of research are also employed in health services and systems research. As discussed in the preface, the authors of this book firmly believe that a public health evaluation framework, based upon a program theory and 'logic model', offers by far the best evaluation approach to the assessment of the medical and public health response to disasters.

At this point it is useful to differentiate evaluation studies from epidemiological studies of disasters. While both types of studies may use similar data collection methods (interviews, medical records review, observation, etc.), the purpose and scope for each approach is different. Evaluation studies should be designed to focus on the operation of the entire response system, as each component functions over time, within a structure–process–outcomes frame-work, often including costs. Disaster epidemiology is typically focused on documenting the extent and causes of injury or death of the victims of a dis-aster, and the health-related effects of the disaster on the population affected, often followed over time.

Scientific evaluative research is based upon two very simple ideas. First, sci-entific methods can be used to assess the process of implementation and the outcomes and effectiveness of any health or human service organization or pro-gram (often referred to as an intervention). Secondly, people, programs, and organizations can evolve and adapt in a way that is planned and increasingly responsive to the needs of society if they become 'self-assessing' and attempt to learn from past experience.

Origins of Evaluative Research

In the late 1960s and early 1970s significant financial support for evalu-ation studies became available in the United States with the passage of 'Great Society' programs such as Medicare, Medicaid, Model Cities, Head Start, and the Emergency Medical Services Act (1973). The legislation that authorized each of these programs required that program evaluation be conducted to as-sess the operation and the resulting effects of each. With each of these, major national legislative initiatives funds were provided to conduct evaluation studies.

The mandate to conduct evaluation and the availability of money, in turn, drew the attention of academic researchers such as Edward Suchman, whose landmark book, 'Evaluative Research', published in 1967, described a compre-hensive framework and methods for scientific program evaluation (Suchman, 1967). Suchman was the first social scientist to describe, in a book, a compre-hensive scientific framework and a set of methods for conducting evaluation studies. His clearly written text and coherent model were rapidly adopted by academics, health administrators, health services researchers, and policy-makers who quickly began to apply the concepts and methods he described to design and implement evaluation studies throughout the United States. Interestingly, Suchman's book was reprinted seven times—without change. It was clearly a 'best seller' due in great part to its timeliness and the clarity and simplicity with which he presented a somewhat complex set of concepts and methods.

However, it became clear rather quickly that the huge initial cohort of evalu-ation studies while produced with great enthusiasm, if even read, tended to remain unused and therefore had little impact upon policy or practice. This unfortunate state of affairs motivated another social scientist, Michael Quinn Patton, to supplement Suchman's approach in a quite important way.

Patton's cogent insights about our inherent human fears of evaluation and the widespread human resistance to change led him to suggest a way to modify these barriers to evaluation by involving key 'stakeholders' in what he labeled a 'utilization-focused' approach. Patton's model can be thought of as complementary to the framework elaborated by Suchman. Patton's approach was designed to increase the likelihood that evaluation findings would be used to improve both the planning and outcomes of human service programs (Patton, 1997).

In addition to the elaboration by Suchman, Patton, and other methodologists of a scientific paradigm for evaluation, the availability of funding for evaluation provided the impetus for academics and members of the many 'Think Tanks' that were formed in the 1970s and beyond to become active participants in the conduct of evaluation studies and to further refine the scientific methodology for evaluation.

As a result, the specialty of evaluation has developed rapidly since the 1960s. In addition to Suchman and Patton, scholars from other social/behavioral science disciplines, and from the human service professions of public health, medicine, social work, and education, have advanced the methodological rigor of evaluation studies. Among the other early evaluation scientists were Cook and Campbell (Cook and Campbell, 1979), whose highly impactful contribution was to identify and describe a number of 'quasi-experimental' designs that could be used to conduct evaluation studies when true experimental (randomized controlled) conditions cannot be achieved. Scriven (1967) contributed to the philosophical underpinnings of the newly emerging specialty of evaluation by differentiating between 'formative' (process-focused) and 'summative' (outcome-focused) evaluation.

Lincoln and Guba (1985), Patton (1990), Miles and Huberman (2014), and Steckler and Linnan (2002) all developed methods to improve the application of qualitative approaches to evaluation.

In addition, Avedis Donabidian (1980) described methods for the application of the basic evaluation concepts of structure, process, and outcome to the evaluation of medical care. Carol Weiss (1972) made highly important clarifications to the emerging scientific framework in her discussions of the political nature of evaluation and by highlighting (with others writing at the time) the importance of what came to be known as 'process evaluation'.

Formed in 1972, the American Evaluation Association (AEA) is a national professional association whose membership has grown rapidly in the decades since its formation. It is currently the largest association of evaluation scientists, although evaluation associations patterned after it have been formed in other countries. In the early 1990s, the AEA promulgated evaluation standards and a code of ethics. Moreover, the AEA has become an international forum for scientific discussion and scholarship. The society has organized international scientific meetings for evaluation scientists. Also, a global network, EvalPartners, has been formed whose purpose is to disseminate information about evaluation methods and to encourage more use of scientific evaluation in all the institutions of 'civil society' (Donaldson et al., 2015) globally. Fortunately, it is now possible to identify and engage with evaluation specialists in more than 70 countries.

However, it is clear that the impact of evaluation has not been equally experienced throughout the domain of human services including public health and medicine; medical and public health systems have remained resistant to the routine application of the advances that have occurred in the development of evaluation as a specialized domain of scientific knowledge and practice. Nonetheless, evaluation scientists and scholars continue to work to increase the scientific rigor of evaluation studies conducted in real-world contexts, develop innovative ways of using mixed-methods designs and methodologies, develop an overarching theory of evaluation science that integrates the various existing schools of thought, and apply the most advanced and exacting methods, when appropriate, from several scientific disciplines. At the present time, a sufficient foundation of methodology exists to enable evaluation science to make significant contributions to the field of disaster preparedness and response.

A Definition of Scientific Evaluation

Edward Suchman, author of the aforementioned 'Evaluative Research', the first book that contains a broad comprehensive framework for scientific evaluation, has defined program evaluation as: 'the general process of judging the worth or value of a program or activity'. A 'program' may be thought of as a 'set of resources and activities directed toward one or more common goals'.

> In our approach we will make a distinction between 'evaluations' and 'evaluative research'. The former will be used in a general way as referring to the social process of making judgements of worth.... it does not require any systematic procedures for marshaling and presenting objective evidence to support the judgement. 'Evaluative research' on the other hand, will be restricted to the utilization of scientific research methods and techniques for the purpose of making an evaluation. In this sense,

> 'evaluative' becomes an adjective specifying a type of research and 'evaluative research' refers to those procedures for collecting and analyzing data which increase the possibility for 'proving' the worth of some social activity.
>
> (Suchman, 1967)

Suchman's distinction between evaluation and evaluative research forms the fundamental underpinning for this book. In this volume, when we use the terms evaluation science or evaluative research, we are referring to the process of using scientific methods to determine the 'value or worth' of the medical and public health response to disasters. Evaluation science is defined as the body of scientific concepts, methods, and analytic approaches used by evaluators. Evaluative research is the process of applying evaluation science to determine the value or worth of a social program (also referred to as an intervention) whose intent is to improve human health or well-being.

A slightly modified definition of scientific evaluation has been offered by Patton who defined program evaluation as:

> the systematic collection of information about the activities, characteristics and outcomes of programs to make judgments about the program, improve program effectiveness and/or inform decisions about future programming. Utilization-focused program evaluation ... is evaluation done for and with specific ... users.
>
> (Patton, 1997)

However Patton was deeply concerned, and rightly so, about the reality that evaluation studies were having little impact towards the goal of improving health programs and policy decisions. This was especially troubling in that by the end of the 1970s, huge amounts of money were being spent on program evaluations. One of his many important contribution to evaluation science was the suggestion that key 'stakeholders' be involved in each evaluation study, from the design stage to the preparation of findings and recommendations. In so doing, he reasoned, each evaluation study was more likely to be used by those who had the power to implement recommendations that were offered at the completion of an evaluation study.

> By the end of the 1960s, it was becoming clear that evaluations of Great Society social programs were largely ignored or politicized. The Utopian hopes for a scientific and rational society had somehow failed to be realized.
>
> (Patton, 1997)

Patton was hardly alone in expressing concern about the reality that little was changing as a result of the great societal investment in evaluation studies; many evaluators, along with officials of organizations that had provided funding for evaluations, were expressing the same concern throughout the 1970s.

However, it was primarily Patton who most forcefully challenged and altered the prevailing paradigm for the conduct of evaluation studies by conceptualizing and providing a strong argument for a 'utilization-focused framework' which involved the extensive participation of key stakeholders throughout the evaluation process. His approach has been widely adopted by organizations and evaluators globally.

Differentiation of Research, Quality Improvement, and Program Evaluation

In the interest of further clarifying and defining the domain of evaluation science, it is useful to consider some important differences and similarities among three different but interrelated activities, namely scientific research, quality improvement, and scientific program evaluation. Staff members of the Nova Scotia Research Fund have prepared a set of guiding questions that may be applied to differentiate program evaluation from research quality improvement. They have approached the task by posing a set of definitional questions that might be asked. We offer a modified version of their work in Table 2.1.

As can be seen from the information presented in Table 2.1, the specialties of Quality Improvement and Program Evaluation have been created because they are able to address different questions and societal needs than those of traditional clinical or basic research. In addition, they are able to answer different kinds of questions than are typically addressed by more fundamental research and they are fully embedded in the context in which they are carried out.

Evaluation Perspectives

A scientific approach to evaluation requires (1) a general conceptual framework that can be applied to design each evaluation study; (2) rigorous methods for designing the study and for data collection and analysis which provide valid and reliable data; and (3) systematic analysis and interpretation of evaluative data in order to offer judgments about the quality of the intervention program and recommendations for program improvement that are derived directly from the findings of the study. In addition, it is widely accepted today that the organized participation of a 'stakeholder group' at all key steps in the evaluation process is an essential element of an evaluation study because such participation is expected to increase the likelihood that the evaluation findings will be used to improve program performance.

Table 2.1 Differentiation of research, quality improvement, and program evaluation

	Research	Quality improvement	Program evaluation
What is the purpose of your project?	To generate new knowledge, which is generalizable to the wider population. Generalizable knowledge consists of facts, theories, principles, or relationships, which can be corroborated using scientific methods.	To improve internal processes, practices, costs, or productivity for a specific intervention (i.e. determine how *this* intervention affected *this* participant group in *this* setting).	To inform decisions, identify improvements (i.e. formative evaluation), and provide information about the success of programs (i.e. summative evaluation) according to predefined goals and objectives.
Will you be using an experimental or quasi-experimental design?	Yes, either of these may be used.	No.	Quasi-experimental; non-experimental design; qualitative, quantitative, and mixed-methods designs and analysis may be used.
How will you handle extraneous variables?	Try to control or measure them.	Acknowledge them, but do not try to interfere with them. They are part of any real life experience.	Use multiple lines of evidence to answer evaluation questions related to program implementation and outcomes.
How will you analyze the data?	With inferential statistics to test for significant differences, descriptive statistics, or a qualitative methodology that can compare and contrast qualitative data.	With descriptive statistics that demonstrate change/trends.	Quantitative (inferential and descriptive analysis) and qualitative data and analysis may be used.
What do you plan to do with your findings? How will they be applied?	Disseminate findings as widely as possible to increase the body of scientific knowledge by publishing or presenting for others within the discipline.	Communicate findings within the organization primarily by providing specific feedback to decision makers responsible for managing the practice. Findings may also be published with organizational approval.	Communicate findings within the program and organization primarily by providing specific feedback to those who commissioned the evaluation. Findings may also be published with organizational approval.

Table 2.1 Continued

	Research	Quality improvement	Program evaluation
Is Research Ethics Board approval required?	Yes—an ethics board approval is usually also required for publication in a research journal.	No.	No.
How will your findings change practice/ policy?	Findings will contribute to scientific body of knowledge which collectively adds to evidence that will inform practice/policy.	Will change practice in my setting immediately.	Will improve program design and implementation (i.e. redefine target population), and identify efficient practices, unintended benefits, and threats.

Data from *Nova Scotia Health Authority Research Fund Guide* (Revised October 2018). Nova Scotia Health Authority Research Fund. Appendix A: Guiding Questions to Distinguish Research, Program Evaluation and Quality Improvement, pp. 23–26.

We believe some of the variations one finds in the scientific evaluation literature, and at times confusion, comes from a failure to differentiate the various types and purposes of evaluation studies. Øvretveit's classification of evaluation perspectives, as described in the following paragraphs, is quite useful as a basis for definitional clarity.

'An evaluation perspective both "sees" and "focuses" on certain aspects of an evaluation and on its consequences' (Øvretveit, 1998). The perspectives from which evaluation studies are designed and carried out, can be classified essentially into one of three groups: (1) managerial; (2) economic; and (3) experimental, although more than one perspective may be included in a single evaluation.

Managerial

According to Øvretveit, managerial evaluations are devised and carried out so that managers can monitor or improve performance[1]. They are used to assess accountability, efficiency, appropriateness, safety, effectiveness, and value (benefits) of the services provided. They aim to improve the intervention with strong input from the user(s) of the evaluation. There are at least three types of managerial evaluations: (1) routine monitoring; (2) special monitoring, usually

[1] Øvretveit, following Patton has identified a fourth perspective which they have labelled 'developmental'. We include the developmental perspective in our managerial category while recognizing this varies somewhat from Øvretveit and Patton's use of the concept. Refer to Patton, M.Q. (2011) *Developmental Evaluation*. New York, NY: The Guilford Press.

externally conducted; and (3) comprehensive evaluations that assess the extent to which a program or intervention meets the needs of patients or a population. Managerial studies have substantial relevance for disaster medicine. They are more and more drawing upon a 'program theory' as described in a 'logic model' and they almost always use a 'mixed-methods' approach.

Economic

Economic evaluations focus on the quantity of resources that are consumed by a particular response effort, and/or to quantify the consequences of an action, usually in terms of economic costs. This perspective always assumes that the resources consumed could have been used for another purpose. There are six types of economic evaluation: (1) cost description that allows explicit or implicit comparison of costs of one or more elements of a response; (2) cost minimization that assumes differences in outcomes and calculates the cost of each alternative in an attempt to identify the alternative with the lowest cost; (3) cost effectiveness that compares the costs of different ways of achieving the same outputs/effects; (4) cost utility in which states of health associated with outcomes are valued relative to one another; (5) cost benefit in which benefits in terms of expense are compared as to their worth; and (6) opportunity costs since many resources can only be used once, forcing prioritization (Øvretveit 1998). Economic evaluations are used to evaluate treatments, services, and health policies, but only infrequently are used for organizational interventions.

Experimental and Quasi-experimental Perspectives

Experimental studies are directed at defining cause–effect relationships and are used to define the impact of specific interventions. Currently, such studies have limited application in the study of disasters and the responses to them. Their greatest application today is in comparing specific treatments provided to groups of patients, for example the evaluation of different types of psychiatric treatments provided in the acute, mid-, or long-term phases of the disaster, different types of field anesthesia, use of prophylactic antibiotics during a disaster, and the like. They are also useful when examining the capacity of varying types of structures (buildings, bridges, roads, etc.) to withstand the extreme forces experienced in a disaster such as an earthquake, tornado, or hurricane.

However, important information can be derived from the use of quasi-experimental studies in the identification of probable cause and effect. Quasi-experimental studies include longitudinal studies in which patients serve as their own controls in a before and after design, case-controlled studies, and observational studies using either crossover designs or longitudinal designs. Non-randomized, controlled trials are similar in most respects to randomized studies, but the groups being compared cannot be randomized. Therefore, the internal validity of quasi-experimental studies is not as great as for randomized studies as there is greater likelihood for bias and confounding variables to be introduced. Again, it is important to emphasize that experimental studies of specific interventions currently have little application in the evaluation of responses to disasters.

The identification of these perspectives is highly useful because once an evaluation team has clarity about the purpose of the evaluation (either to improve the implementation and management of an existing or new program or to develop a new 'evidence-based' intervention), it becomes clear as to which design options are appropriate. If the goal of the evaluation is to develop and test a new intervention then an experimental approach is the desirable framework. If, however, one is assessing an existing program, as is the case with disaster evaluations, then an approach based upon a 'program theory/logic model' is the preferred design option.

Standards for Evaluation Studies

In 1994, a broadly representative committee of evaluation scientists published a set of 'standards for evaluation'. The 30 evaluation standards were grouped into four general categories as shown in Box 2.1. As described by the committee:

> The standards ... call for evaluations that have four features. These are utility, feasibility, propriety, and accuracy ... Their rationale is that an evaluation should not be done at all if there is no prospect for it being useful to some audience (utility). Second, it should not be done if it is not feasible to conduct in political, practical, or cost effectiveness terms. Third ... it should (not) be done if ... not conducted fairly and ethically (propriety). Finally ... we can turn to the difficult matters of technical accuracy.
>
> (Patton, 1997)

These standards represent an important step in the development of scientific evaluation in that they form the basis for the professionalization of evaluation as it is practiced today. With professionalism has come a code of ethics and formal training in universities for those who choose to pursue careers as program evaluation specialists. They have been approved by the American National Standards Institute (ANSI Standard No. ISEE.PR 1994). They have also been endorsed by the American Evaluation Association and numerous other professional organizations, globally.

Box 2.1 Standards for evaluation

Utility

Ensure that an evaluation (study) will serve the information needs of users (stakeholders).

Feasibility

Ensure that an evaluation (study) will be realistic, prudent, diplomatic, and frugal.

Propriety

Ensure that an evaluation (study) will be conducted legally, ethically, and with due regard for the welfare of those involved in the evaluation as well as those affected by the results.

Accuracy

Ensure that an evaluation will reveal and convey technically [accurate] information about … the program being evaluated.

Reproduced from Patton, M.Q., *Utilization-Focused Evaluation: The New Century Text*, p. 17. Copyright © 1996, SAGE College, with permission.

General Model for Program Evaluations that are Focused on Issues of Management and Implementation

A general model for scientific evaluation is shown in Figure 2.1. The steps shown are drawn from an evaluation model that was developed by the US Centers for Disease Control and Prevention in 1999, with our minor modifications. This model is primarily intended to be applied when the purpose is to learn lessons in order to improve the structure, process, and outcomes of a medical or public program (often referred to as 'the intervention'), what we have labeled earlier as a 'managerial evaluation'. This type of evaluation has a different focus than controlled experimental evaluation studies, whose primary goal is to develop evidence-based interventions.

In the US Centers for Disease Control (CDC) model, program evaluation should begin with the engagement of a group of persons who have a strong interest in the outcome of the evaluation (stakeholders) because they may have paid for some aspects of the program, or have been affected by it, or because they have public policy or programmatic responsibility. The stakeholders, working with evaluation scientists, prepare the evaluation questions and evaluation

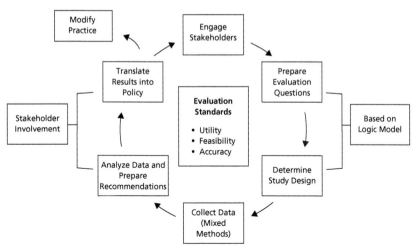

Figure 2.1 Major steps in program evaluation showing feedback process.

design. The questions and design are obtained from a logic model which is a theory of how the preparedness and intervention system should work. The evaluation team members then collect data and prepare a preliminary report of findings and recommendations which is then reviewed by the entire stakeholder group. The stakeholder comments are addressed by the evaluation team members who then prepare a final report which should contain a description of the evaluation methods used, data, findings, and conclusions. As summarized by Donaldson et al.:

> Simply stated, evaluators work with stakeholders to develop a common understanding of how a program is presumed to solve the problem(s) of interest; to formulate and prioritize key evaluation questions; and then decide how best to gather credible evidence to answer those questions.
>
> (Donaldson et al., 2015)

Some Distinguishing Features of Evaluation Research

Although evaluation studies use concepts and methods drawn from the social, behavioral, and public health disciplines, the field itself focuses primarily on practical programmatic issues (managerial) or upon the development and testing of interventions (experimental). Evaluation scientists try to determine which programs/activities/services are effective and which are not effective. They specify the indicators and standards by which these questions may be addressed and they often attempt to determine the costs associated with the achieved results.

Scientific evaluation studies draw upon the full range of research designs available to researchers; however, the organization and conduct of managerial evaluative studies differ from that of research using experimental designs such as randomized controlled trials. When experimental or quasi-experimental designs are not employed, the reasons may include the following: (1) randomized controlled trials are not feasible, such as in the case of evaluating the provision of pre-hospital care under a variety of constraints as occur in disasters; (2) program evaluation is often not concerned with generalizability as it is assumed that community-level interventions are context-sensitive or dependent; therefore matters of generalizability are of less concern; (3) the involved evaluator may provide feedback to program stakeholders who together may recommend changes in program operation or structure; (4) *non*-standardization of program components and implementation across sites is most often the situation encountered when evaluating community-based single or multi-site programs; (5) information reaching a decision-maker too late to inform the decision process sometimes results from an overly elegant study design mismatched with time and funding constraints.

A form of evaluation that can at times be useful in disaster evaluation studies is a process that compares the results of an intervention with a set of 'preexisting standards'. The standards can refer to both outcomes and outputs. Community-based disaster preparedness and response teams may establish standards based upon past experience or, simply, their subjective sense of what constitutes a desirable process or outcome.

Here the question becomes, Did the expected changes occur? Or, were the desired outcomes achieved? Or, was the desired response activity implemented within the planned timeframe? The outputs and outcomes are often compared to pre-established standards, for example a 5–10 minute window to get to a disaster scene when using geographic positioning systems (GPS) technology; or, 'Search and rescue should begin within first hour.'

In this type of assessment, no control group is used. If there is no impact, or if the impact is less than the standard, changes in intermediate steps could be suggested. Regardless of the inability to causally link the program activities to observed changes, sufficient confidence may ensue to conclude that program objectives are/are not being met by the intervention that has been reviewed. At times elements of the disaster response effort can be counterproductive or unintended and, unfortunately, this is not uncommon. For that reason the process evaluation component should always include questions that search for and describe counterproductive as well as productive elements of the response.

Mixed-methods Designs

As the conceptual and design framework for the conduct of scientific evaluations evolved during the 1970s and 1980s, a methodological clarification called 'mixed methods' emerged. The proponents of mixed methods, following the philosophical principle that 'There are many windows to the truth', found value in both 'naturalistic' and 'positivist' approaches to the conduct of science. The original mixed-methods designs were based upon the process of 'triangulation'. Triangulation refers to a process whereby several methods are used to obtain data about a variable or set of variables. For example, the scientist could observe a behavior, ask others what they saw, then draw information from written records and compare the observations. If they converge, more confidence is reached in the conclusions drawn from the findings.

> The most common and well-known approach to mixing methods is the Triangulation Design. The purpose of this design is 'to obtain different but complementary data on the same topic' … to best understand the research problem. The intent in using this design is to bring together the different strengths and non-over lapping weaknesses of quantitative methods … with those of qualitative methods.
>
> (Patton, 1990)

The basic triangulation design has evolved into several variants, namely (1) 'convergence model'; (2) 'data transformation model'; (3) 'validating quantitative data model' and (4) the 'multilevel mixed-methods' model.

In the 'convergence model' the researcher collects and analyzes quantitative and qualitative data separately on the same phenomena and then the different results are converged, for example with survey data and focus group data. In the 'data transformation model' the data are collected using separate methods but one data set is transformed so that both data sets are in the same form, either quantitative or qualitative. This transformation allows the analyst to 'mix' or combine the data in the process of analysis. The 'validating quantitative data model' is used when researchers want to validate and expand on quantitative findings. This can be done, for instance, by adding open-ended questions to a structured quantitative survey.

One more variant of a mixed-methods approach is 'multilevel research'. In a multilevel model, 'different methods (quantitative and qualitative) are used to address different levels within a system. The findings from each level are merged into one overall interpretation' (Tashakkori and Teddlie, 1998; Creswell, 2006). The key word here is 'interpretation' in that the analysis process requires that the analysis will tell a full story of the intervention and its outcomes after applying both quantitative and qualitative data to the research questions of interest. It is the 'multilevel mixed-methods' model that we suggest is the most appropriate approach to evaluating the medical and public health response to a disaster.

Barriers to Evaluation

Unfortunately, there are many barriers to the conduct of evaluation studies and these may prevent the initiation of an evaluation, or they may prevent change from happening even though the research indicates that change will make things better. Some of these barriers may seem inappropriate, but nevertheless they may be erected to block any change that may be suggested by the stake-holders and evaluation team. Some of the more commonly encountered barriers are discussed.

Human

- National pride in how things are done and have been done in the past. Often, a national mandate may go with the current way things are done. Politically, maintaining the status quo may have an advantage because effecting change may be perceived as a weakness or an indication of past failure.
- Recommendations may be viewed as criticism, and criticism is seldom taken lightly and may even be considered a serious threat to the organization or system being evaluated. The recommendations may not fit with the culture, and hence may be rejected.
- Some organizations may have a vested interest in continuing along the current lines. They may have secondary motives for the assistance that is provided.
- Funding may not be available to implement the suggested changes.

Technical

- There exists a lack of experience and/or training about disaster medicine/ health disasters and public health on the part of the evaluation team.
- Data collection barriers are extreme.

Thus, the ability to create change in an organization, or in public policy, may depend upon the presence of persons in an organization who have a high degree of personal experience who also have a high level of experience and respect.

It is likely that some of the resistance to change can be diminished through the provision of education about the true nature of evaluation studies. If it is known and accepted by the members of the organization being evaluated that positive aspects will be highlighted and that key stakeholders will be involved, resistance may be lessened. Hopefully, the approach described in this book will serve as a basis for the development and implementation of disaster evaluation studies that will counter most if not all of these barriers.

Basic Assumptions for Evaluation Studies

We believe that all evaluation studies should be based upon an underlying set of basic values and assumptions. These are:

- Evaluation is a basic function of management.
- Evaluative findings and recommendations should be used when making decisions about change in health intervention programs or projects.
- The methods used to evaluate a program or project should be fully understood by the individuals who are being evaluated.
- All individuals who have a stake in the results of an evaluation study should be members of the 'stakeholder group' that works with the evaluation team.
- Evaluation should be used for positive growth and improvement; it should thus be viewed as a constructive management tool.
- Evaluations should be balanced in that good performance should be recognized as well as areas for improvement.
- The least expensive evaluation study that will meet scientific standards and answer the questions of the stakeholder group should be used so that scarce resources are not wasted.
- Evaluation research relies upon the scientific method and standards, but these should recognize the political, ethical, and cultural context for each study.
- Scientific evaluation is only one tool of management. Management judgments based upon experience and intuition are still of value when programmatic or policy decisions are made.

We believe that these broad and fundamental assumptions, and the values embedded in them, underlie all scientific evaluation studies (Ricci and Nolan, 2009).

Summary

The specialty of evaluative research has developed rapidly since the 1960s when the first book which described a comprehensive framework and methodology for evaluation science was written by Edward Suchman, an academic social psychologist. The passage of a large body of social legislation in the United States in the mid-1960s brought an infusion of governmental and foundation money and interest to support the fledgling specialty. This support brought about a large increase in the number of comprehensive and rigorous evaluative studies, even more funding, continued development, and refinement of the conceptual and methodological underpinnings for evaluation and, finally, the professionalization of evaluation as a specialty within the human service professions.

Acknowledgment

The extract from WHO 2015 is reprinted from *Ethics in Epidemics, Emergencies and Disasters: Research Surveillance and Patient Care*, p. 29, © World Health Organization, 2015. The extract from Patton, M.Q., *Qualitative Evaluation and Research Methods*. Newbury Park, CA: Sage Publications. Copyright © 1990, Sage Publications, is reproduced here with permission. The extract from Suchman, E.A., *Evaluative Research*, p. 75. New York: Russell Sage Foundation. Copyright © 1967, Russell Sage Foundation, is reproduced here with permission. The extract from Patton, M.Q., *Utilization-focused evaluation: The new century text*, p. 17. Copyright © 1997 SAGE College, is reproduced here with permission.

References

CDC. (1999). Centers for Disease Control and Prevention Framework for Program Evaluation in Public Health. *Morbidity and Mortality Weekly Report*. **48**:RR11.

Chan, M. (2013). *WHO Evaluation Practice Handbook*. Geneva, Switzerland: WHO Press, p. v.

Cook, T.D. and Campbell, D. (1979). *Quasi Experimentation; Design and Analysis Issues for Field Settings*. Chicago, IL: Rand McNally.

Creswell, J.W. and Plano Clark, V.L. (2006). *Designing and Conducting Mixed Methods Research*. Thousand Oaks, CA: Sage Publications.

Donabidian, A. (1980). *The Definition of Quality and Approaches to Its Assessment*. Ann Arbor, MI: Health Administration Press.

Donaldson, S.I., Christie, E.A., and Mark, M.M., eds. (2015). *Credible and Actionable Evidence*, 2nd ed. Thousand Oaks, CA: Sage Publications.

Lincoln, Y.S. and Guba, E.G. (1985). *Naturalistic Inquiry*. Newbury Park, CA: Sage Publications.

Miles, M. and Huberman, M. (1994). *Qualitative Data Analysis*, 3rd ed. Thousand Oaks, CA: Sage Publications.

Nova Scotia Health Authority Research Fund Guide (Revised October 2018). Nova Scotia Health Authority Research Fund. Appendix A: Guiding Questions to Distinguish Research, Program Evaluation and Quality Improvement, pp. 23–26.

Øvretveit, J. (1998). *Evaluating Health Interventions*. Milton Keynes, UK: Open University Press, pp. 34–36.

Patton, M.Q. (1990). *Qualitative Evaluation and Research Methods*. Newbury Park, CA: Sage Publications.

Patton, M.Q. (1997). *Utilization Focused Evaluation*, 3rd ed. Thousand Oaks, CA: Sage Publications, pp. 17, 23.

Ricci, E.M. and Nolan, B. (2009). The future integration of scientific evaluation in project management. In: Cleland, D. and Bidanda, B., eds. *Project Management Circa 2025*, 1st ed. Newtown Square, PA: Project Management Institute, p. 203.

Scriven, M. (1967). The methodology of evaluation. In: Gagne, R.W. and Scriven, M., eds. *Perspectives of Curriculum Evaluation*, 1st ed. Chicago, IL: Rand McNally, pp. 39–83.

Steckler, A.B. and Linnan, L. (2002). *Process Evaluation*. San Francisco, CA: Josey Bass and Sons, Inc.

Suchman, E.A. (1967). *Evaluative Research*. New York, NY: Russell Sage Foundation, p. 75.

Tashakkori, A. and Teddlie, C. (1998). *Handbook of Mixed Methods in Social and Behavioral Research*. Thousand Oaks, CA: Sage Publications.

Weiss, C. (1972). *Evaluation Research: Methods for Assessing Program Effectiveness*. Englewood Cliffs, NJ: Prentice Hall, Inc.

WHO. (2015). *Ethics in Epidemics, Emergencies and Disasters: Research Surveillance and Patient Care*. Geneva, Switzerland: World Health Organization, p. 29.

Further reading

Denzin, N.K. and Lincoln, Y.S., eds. (2011). *The Sage Handbook of Qualitative Research*. Thousand Oaks, CA: Sage Publications.

Patton, M.Q. (2008). *Utilization Focused Evaluation*, 4th ed. Thousand Oaks, CA: Sage Publications.

Patton, M.Q. (2011). *Essentials of Utilization Focused Evaluation*. Thousand Oaks, CA: Sage Publications.

Shortell, S.M. and Richardson, W.C. (1978). *Health Program Evaluation*. Saint Louis, MO: C.V. Mosby Company.

US Department of Health and Human Services, Centers for Disease Control and Prevention, Office of Strategy and Innovation. (2011). *Introduction to Program Evaluation for Public Health Programs: A Self Study Guide*. Atlanta, GA: Centers for Disease Control and Prevention.

Chapter 3

Introduction to a Model for Disaster Evaluation

Keypoints

In this chapter we move to a discussion of the determination of objectives for a disaster evaluation study and the rationale behind the design and use of a logic model. Logic models are now widely used throughout the domain of public health as a tool for both designing and evaluating health programs (typically referred to as 'interventions'). This chapter is offered as a general introduction to the detailed discussion of eight steps for conducting a disaster evaluation as presented in Part 2 of this Field Manual. The selection of two key components of our general evaluation framework, 'evaluation objectives' and 'program theory/logic model' for further discussion, is to highlight the centrality and importance of these ideas and concepts for scientific evaluations.

A disaster response evaluation study is defined as a scientific endeavor to gather evidence to elucidate the causes, circumstances, risk factors and extent of human and health system damage during the life cycle of a disaster. A major goal of such studies is the conduct of assessments of the quality of life saving and life supporting actions implemented during and after a disaster in order to improve the response to future disasters.
(Sundnes et al., 2014)

The definition of disaster preparedness and response evaluation by Sundnes et al. defines and bounds our focus in this Field Manual. The definition has evolved from the meetings and work of the aforementioned Task Force on Quality Control of Disaster Management (TFQCDM), an international group of physicians and scientists who have worked since 2001 to improve the medical and public health aspects of disaster response, in part through improved evaluation (Sundnes 2014).

Why Is a Scientific Evaluation Framework Based on a Program Theory and Logic Model, the Best Framework for Disaster Evaluation?

A logic model, sometimes thought of as a diagram of a theory of how a program should work, is a key building block of modern scientific evaluations. It is especially useful in situations such as large disasters where controlled experimental designs are not feasible. Today, public health students receive training in how to prepare logic models and then use them as a key tool for management and evaluation.

As previously noted, we are making the case in this book that a scientific evaluation framework is really the best framework for disaster evaluation. It is the best approach because it is based on a program theory, as described in a logic model, which guides the evaluation to measure each component of the logic model. This process can then lead to a comprehensive explanation of why the intended outcomes of the disaster response were or were not reached. No other framework is as comprehensive and as targeted on the key variables needed for a description and explanation of the actual performance of a health intervention as is the approach we are describing in the field manual.

There are, however, other models in current use for disaster evaluation studies. The discipline of *epidemiology* provides surveillance methods which can be a useful component of a comprehensive evaluation. *Social science*-based studies are usually not intended to be evaluative, although the methods used in social science research certainly have utility in evaluation. Social science-based approaches have other purposes, mainly to offer a deep description of what occurred during and following the disaster event and an explanation of the consequences of the disaster upon the affected community and upon the lives of those affected by the disaster. These studies typically focus on broad contextual factors and are thus valuable in providing a panorama of effects. *Engineering models* are usually focused on a question or problem subject to engineering intervention (e.g. why buildings or roads or bridges, etc., failed to survive the force of a disaster; how buildings could be constructed to better withstand the forces evoked by disasters of various types).

However, we contend that it is only a scientific evaluation framework, based upon a program theory as described in a logic model, that offers a comprehensive approach for scientific evaluation of the medical and public health response to disasters. This approach leads to 'theory-based evaluations'. Why are theory-based evaluations more useful and stronger methodologically than those that are not based on a program theory? The following statement by Fitz-Gibbon and Morris provides some clarity in that they explain the linkage among the variables contained in the theory of how an intervention is expected to work to achieve the desired effects (outcomes) by specifying hypothesized relations between activities and outcomes:

> What do we mean by theory-based evaluation? A theory based evaluation of a program is one in which the selection of program features is determined by an explicit conceptualization of the program in terms of a theory which attempts to explain how the program produces the desired effects.
>
> (Fitz-Gibbon and Morris, 1996)

Fitz-Gibbon and Morris state further that the essential component of a program theory is the specification of a set of causal relationships. That there is a causal relationship between a process (A) and an outcome (B). The logic model framework is the most widely used format for providing a detailed delineation of how an intervention process is connected to the expected outcomes, especially one that involves many activities and outcomes. This way of 'framing' the relationships, which a scientific evaluation should be designed to uncover, can be traced to the work of Suchman (1967). Although Suchman did not use the term logic model he clearly described a way of conceptualizing evaluation studies that is totally consistent with the current definition of a logic model design.

The preparation of a logic model can bring order and focus to an evaluation in that the main variables of interest are clearly revealed as are the expected relationships between the intervention process and expected outcomes.

Benefits Derived from Using a Theory-based/ Logic Model Evaluation Framework for Disaster Evaluation Studies

There are many benefits that can result from the application of an evaluation framework, based upon a logic model that describes the medical and public health response to a disaster. Among these benefits are:

♦ Since the evaluation framework provides the most comprehensive approach to assess the structure and function of the disaster preparedness and response system it can be used to address a wide range of evaluative questions.

- ◆ A theory-based evaluation framework provides the most structured and comprehensive approach to the assessment.

- ◆ An evaluation framework, with its accompanying concepts and methods as described in this volume, has been adopted by the US Centers for Disease Control, the World Health Organization, and Health Systems Research Organizations, internationally, and is therefore widely recognized and supported.

- ◆ A theory-based evaluation framework provides a standardized approach which applies across cultures and disaster types.

- ◆ The logic model design, which is integral to a theory-based evaluation framework, can lead to a standardized approach to the design and implementation of disaster evaluation studies which, in turn, will facilitate comparative analysis across disasters.

- ◆ A standardized theory-based approach to evaluation could facilitate the creation of an international data archive, one goal of which could be to store and catalogue data to be used to arrive at 'best practices' for the medical and public health response to disasters.

Logic Models, Goals, and Objectives for Disaster Evaluation

A widely accepted definition of the term logic model has been provided by the Kellogg Foundation:

> The program logic model is defined as a picture of how your organization does its work – the theory and assumptions underlying the program. A program logic model links the (intended) outcomes (both short term and long term) with program activities/processes and the theoretical assumptions/principles of the program.
>
> (W.K. Kellogg Foundation, 2004)

Moreover, a logic model is one of the most useful conceptual frameworks available to health program planners and evaluation scientists. Its purpose is to describe both the detailed set of activities to be conducted by those who are attempting to 'intervene' in order to ameliorate a societal problem and the expected results of their efforts.

Embedded in every logic model is a set of hypotheses which describe how the intervention program is expected to work, and it should make obvious why the intervention (in our case the medical and public health response) is a rational solution to the problem being addressed.

Logic models are used to design programs of intervention to improve health and to reduce morbidity and mortality. As shown in Figure 3.1, a detailed logic

'if–then'

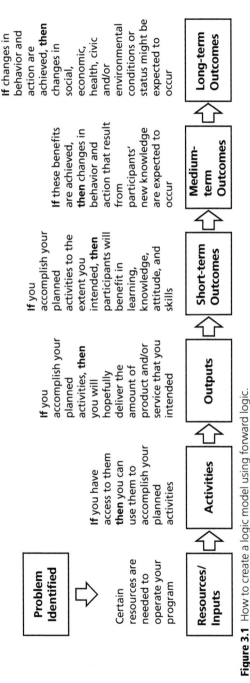

Figure 3.1 How to create a logic model using forward logic.

Reproduced from *Logic Model Development Guide: Using Logic Models to Bring Together Planning, Evaluation, and action* p. 3 Copyright © 1998 by the W.K. Kellogg Foundation.

model clearly identifies the goals, objectives, and activities necessary to reach a set of desired outcomes, the available resources (inputs), the outputs resulting from the programmatic activities, and the short-term and longer-term expected outcomes including the eventual impact on the morbidity and mortality of the target population.

Since a logic model contains a set of hypothesized relationships (either made explicit or implied), it shows the expected (hoped for) outputs and outcomes which can be expressed in the form of a theory of how the response should work. We carry out the evaluation to test the logic model against the reality of the response for each activity and its related outcome. It is certainly possible that some or all of the actual outcomes may be negative; that is, what we had hoped or expected to result is not achieved; however, the reverse is also possible. That is, the response may be so effective that few lives are lost and disaster related injuries are minimal.

In Figure 3.1 we illustrate the thought process that is followed in preparing a logic model. The reader will observe this logic as we apply it later in this Field Manual to design a generalized logic model for disaster evaluation studies.

We find it helpful to differentiate between goals and objectives. Following Sundnes (2014), goals are defined as broad statements that are visionary in nature and not easy to accurately measure; for example, to ease pain and suffering in the population of individuals who live in a disaster area. Objectives are specific statements of expected results. The most useful objectives for planning and evaluation are *s*pecific, *m*easurable, *a*ttainable, *r*esults oriented and usually expressed within a *t*imeframe (SMART). For example: Following a major earthquake all victims will be identified and, if alive, triaged within 48 hours of the event. If the objectives are specific and measurable it is a straightforward next step to establish indicators for the assessment of each.

Furthermore, an evaluation of the medical and public health components of a disaster preparedness and response program could address numerous programmatic and policy objectives, for example to:

- Assess the effectiveness of the public health and medical response in terms of morbidity and mortality reduction in the affected population.
- Assess the potential for further lifesaving and reduction of morbidity during the disaster event.
- Determine how to better organize and implement a relief effort; how to manage during periods of disruption and disorder; identify the criteria by which to allocate resources.
- Develop recommendations for the design and implementation of various pre-event mitigation measures.

- Design, implement, and assess effectiveness of a tabletop, field top, or full field preparedness and response exercise; identify indicators of success and failure.

- Assess the long-term effects of a disaster on individuals and communities.

- Assess preparedness objectives; learn more about hazards and community vulnerabilities germane to the local area or region.

- Design, implement, and refine planning and budgetary procedures so that disaster response operational effectiveness can be balanced with cost efficiency.

A Final Comment about the Utility of a Program Theory for Disaster Evaluation Studies

In the landmark book, *Experimental and Quasi-Experimental Designs for Generalized Causal Inference,* Shadish et al. (2002), in discussing non-experimental alternatives to experimental and quasi-experimental designs, write the following about 'theory-based evaluations'.

> Its origins are in path analysis and causal modelling, traditions that are much older. Although advocates have some differences with each other, basically they all contend that it is useful: (1) to explicate the theory of a treatment by detailing the expected re-lationships among inputs, mediating processes, and short- and long-term outcomes; (2) to measure all the constructs specified in the theory; and (3) to analyse the data to assess the extent to which the postulated relationships actually occurred. For shorter time periods, the available data may address only the first part of a postulated causal chain; but over longer periods the complete model could be involved. Thus, the priority is on highly specific substantive theory, high-quality measurement, and valid analysis of multivariate explanatory processes as they unfold in time.
>
> It (theory-based evaluations) is attractive for several reasons. First, it requires only a treatment group, not a comparison group whose agreement to be in the study might be problematic and whose participation increases research costs. Second, demonstrating a match between theory and data suggests the validity of the causal theory without having to go through a laborious process of explicitly considering alternative explan-ations. Third, it is often impractical to measure distant end points ... theory-specified processes can be used in the interim to inform program staff about effectiveness to date, to argue for more program resources if the program seems to be on theoretical track, to justify claims that the program might be effective in the future on the as-yet-not-assessed distant criteria, and to defend against premature summative evaluations that claim that an intervention is ineffective before it has been demonstrated that the processes necessary for the effect have actually occurred.
>
> (Shadish et al., 2002)

This statement is quite remarkable in that Shadish et al. have been the leading proponents of the use of experimental and quasi-experimental designs to examine the effects of an intervention. Their recognition of the value of theory-based evaluations, and their explication of the underlying logic of such an approach, represents highly credible support for theory-based evaluations, especially in the situation presented by disaster evaluation studies where it is not possible to design and implement controlled experimental or quasi-experimental evaluation projects.

Essential Building Blocks for Disaster Evaluation Studies

In Figure 3.2, we have summarized the disaster evaluation components discussed in Chapters 2 and 3.

Each of the components presented in Figure 3.2 is essential to the design and implementation of a comprehensive evaluation of the medical and public health response to disaster. These components will be used in the eight-step model described in Part 2 of this Field Manual.

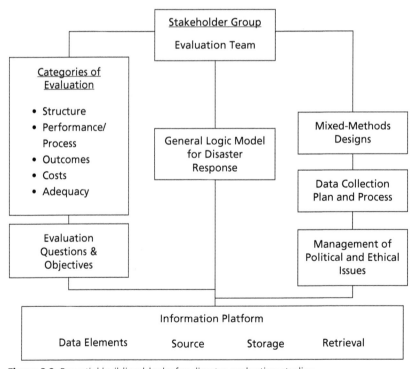

Figure 3.2 Essential building blocks for disaster evaluation studies.

Summary

Owing to their centrality, this chapter has focused upon two key building blocks of our suggested conceptual approach to the design of a disaster evaluation: (1) a logic model, and (2) a clearly stated response system objectives and outcomes. The clear specification of evaluation objectives, response activities, and expected outcomes in the form of a logic model is essential for a theory-based scientific evaluation. The chapter concluded with a diagram showing each of the essential building blocks for the design and implementation of a scientific evaluation that will have sufficient rigor to add to the knowledge base upon which future disaster preparedness and response efforts may be based.

Acknowledgment

The extract from Shadish, W.R., et al., *Experimental and Quasi-Experimental Designs for Generalized Causal Inference*, pp. 501–502. Belmont, CA: Wadsworth Cengage Learning. Copyright © 2002, Cengage Learning, is reproduced here with permission. The extract from Sundnes, K.O. ed., Health Disaster Management: Guidelines for Evaluation And Research in the "Utstein Style". *Scandinavian Journal of Public Health*. 42 (14), pp. 36–47. Copyright © 2014, Sage Publications, is reproduced here with permission.

References

Fitz-Gibbon, C.T. and Morris, L.L. (1996). Theory-based Evaluation. *American Journal of Evaluation*. **17** (2), p. 177.

Shadish, W.R., Cook, T.D., and Campbell, D.T. (2002). *Experimental and Quasi-Experimental Designs for Generalized Causal Inference*. Belmont, CA: Wadsworth Cengage Learning, pp. 501–502.

Suchman, E.A. (1967). *Evaluative Research*. New York, NY: Russell Sage Foundation, p. 84.

Sundnes K.O., ed. (2014). Health Disaster Management: Guidelines for Evaluation and Research in the "Utstein Style". *Scandinavian Journal of Public Health*. **42** (14), p. 38.

W.K. Kellogg Foundation. (Revised 2004). *W.K. Kellogg Foundation Logic Model Development Guide*. Battle Creek, MI: W.K. Kellogg Foundation, p. 3.

Further reading

McLaughlin, J.A. and Jordon, G.B. (1999). Logic Models: A Tool for Telling your Program's Performance Story. *Evaluation and Program Planning*. **22** (1), pp. 62–65.

Wong, D.F., Spencer, C., Boyd, L. et al. (2017). Disaster Metrics: A Comprehensive framework for Disaster Evaluation Typologies. *Prehospital and Disaster Medicine*. **32** (5), pp. 501–517.

Chapter 4

Components of a Disaster Response System

Keypoints

The intent of this chapter is to describe the general framework of emergency public health and emergency medical services operations in disaster events in order to inform the planning and conduct of the evaluation study. The objective of disaster medical and public health response operations is to deliver immediate health care relief to an affected population until 'pre-event' health services can be restored. The functions of the health sector described in this chapter are termed basic societal/support functions or emergency support functions. Each function carries with it a series of activities or interventions; therefore, it seems reasonable to identify and study these activities from the perspective of the user rather than from an event-specific viewpoint. It is important to note that the outcomes or level of performance of these activities be assessed both quantitatively and qualitatively within the context of the larger evaluation study. More importantly, the data collected through systematic evaluation in these cases should be uniformly reported so as to make them generalizable to similar hazard events, thereby facilitating the creation of an 'all-hazards' repository of information on disasters. In this Chapter we describe a generalized disaster response framework, including a 'concept of operations', for the public health and medical components of a disaster response system.

Introduction

We describe a set of functions or activities which are considered essential to temporarily provide relief or support to the medical and public health needs of a population affected by disaster. We refer to this as a 'generalized' model because its components and scope are comprehensive; however, we recognize that not all components may be deployed in every disaster situation due to the type of disaster, the variation in country-specific resources, and in national beliefs about how best to design and implement a response. In Part 2 of this manual we will draw upon these functions to build a logic model and minimum data set for uniform reporting of data in accordance with the 'Utstein Style' (Sundnes, 1999).

The goals of a medical and public health response system in a disaster situation are preparedness, emergency response, and rehabilitation and recovery. The assessment of the health activities implemented in a disaster must include a description of all successes as well as any failures, unwanted and/or unexpected, directly or indirectly, resulting from the response to the event. The findings must be compared to what is known to have existed in the community and health system before the event (pre-event health status). As noted, concomitant changes in the status are not necessarily a result of the intervention. Repeated assessments of the health response can be conducted concurrently (in real time) or at any point during the event and after the event to determine short-term and long-term outcomes of the intervention.

Each intervention should be evaluated as a 'stand-alone' activity in terms of whether its stated objectives were achieved. Other effects (intended or unintended) created by the intervention such as the benefits (impacts) to the affected society accrued from the intervention, the timeliness and efficiency with which it was executed, and the associated costs should also be identified. Box 4.1 presents a comprehensive list of health and medical response activities typically but not always delivered in major disasters.

The Concept of Health and Medical Operations in Disaster

The objectives of the health and medical component of community emergency response aims to (1) provide immediate medical assistance to the ill or injured and address the ongoing health needs of the survivors (safety, food, water, shelter, etc.); (2) quickly restore normal operating conditions and services at health care facilities; and (3) rebuild damaged health infrastructure by taking into account the hazards, their associated risks, and societal vulnerabilities that existed before the event (Sundnes, 2014).

In order to achieve maximum life-saving benefit the disaster response requires effective leadership, management, and communications. The incident management system (IMS) has been developed for this purpose (Stambler and Barbera, 2011). It evolved from the incident command system (ICS), which was based on the work and experiences of the US Forest Fire Brigades (Molino, 2006). The IMS identifies key roles and responsibilities required in large-scale disaster operations (Figure 4.1). The main advantage of the IMS is that it is

Box 4.1 List of emergency public health activities at the community level in response to disasters

- Environmental hazard identification
- Hazards consultation
- Epidemiological services
- Needs identification (health and medical)
- Identification of affected individuals
- Contamination control
- Health (disease) surveillance
- Laboratory specimen collection and analysis
- Infectious disease identification, treatment, and control
- Quarantine/isolation
- Public health information (collection and distribution)
- Risk communication
- Responder safety and health
- Health and medical personnel resources
- Health and medical equipment safety and availability
- Health-related volunteer and donation coordination
- Evacuation Public Health Emergency
- Sheltering
- Special populations need and assistance
- Mass casualty management
- Mortuary services
- Mental/behavioral health care and social services
- Potable water
- Food safety
- Vector control and pest management
- Wastewater and solid-waste management/ disposal
- Building/facility assessment (including structural integrity of critical structures)
- Sanitation/hygiene services
- Restoration of public health programs, services, and infrastructure
- Veterinary services
- Animal rescue/control/shelters
- Long-term community recovery

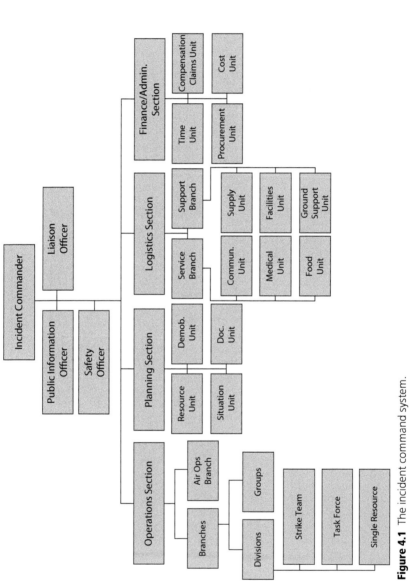

Figure 4.1 The incident command system.

comprehensive, thereby lending itself to an all-hazards approach and applicable to short- and long-term disaster operations, and has been repeatedly tested in actual events.

Major disasters start out as local events and then quickly enlist the aid of higher unaffected geo-political jurisdictions. At the community level, elected officials or their surrogates initially assume the leadership and decision-making role, in partnership with the incident commander selected from among local emergency managers, first responders (fire or police), EMS, or public health services, depending on the type of disaster and the expertise required to lead disaster operations. Once a disaster is declared an emergency operations center (EOC) is activated, thus becoming the location where all disaster operations are coordinated and managed.

The EOC is a physical location (bunker type), see Figure 4.2, ideally equipped with high-tech telecommunications and robust information and communications technology such as satellite telephones and satellite reconnaissance, computers, Internet, television monitors, and integrated geospatial information systems designed to collect information, provide uninterrupted communications, and maintain 'situational awareness' of the event by all participants, everywhere, and at all times (Chan, et al 2004). Disaster managers at the EOC

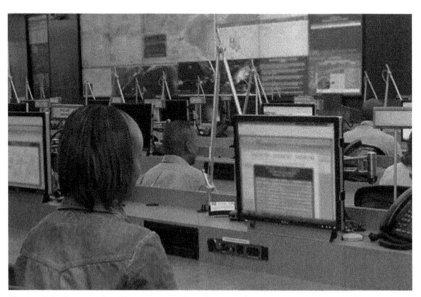

Figure 4.2 Centers for disease control and prevention's emergency operations center (EOC)

work as a team to lead and manage the response. Among the tasks of EOC personnel are:

- dispatch assets and track the progress of the response;
- record and disseminate critical incident information to responders in the field and high-level officials, and keep the public informed;
- coordinate and relieve on-scene commanders of the burden of external co-ordination allowing them to focus on operations;
- conduct periodic needs identification;
- secure necessary supplies, personnel, and other resources.

The effectiveness, robustness, and integrity of the communications system is essential to the success of the disaster response. It includes backup power systems (i.e. battery-powered radios and satellite phones, and electrical generators, etc.) to ensure emergency operations under any conditions.

Once information on the estimated types and numbers of casualties and their location is received by coordinators, resources can be deployed. The time of arrival of rescue units with the injured is received by hospitals, external disaster plans are activated (see hospital disaster plan later). If a surge of casualties exceeds hospital surge capacity, alerts are sent out to neighboring hospitals according to pre-established mutual aid agreements contained in regional disaster response plans. In major sudden-impact disasters such as earthquakes that strike without warning, community capacity to communicate may be hampered requiring state (provincial) or federal (national) assets to be activated and deployed to the disaster zone to aid the local community.

In the United States in the event of a mass or catastrophic disaster the 'National Response Plan' is activated by the President in consultation with the Secretary of the Department of Homeland Security (DHS). In other countries a National Emergency Commission, or similar body, is tasked with implementing a national response (Bissell et al., 1994). The World Health Organization (WHO) provides guidance on the framework for emergency preparedness and governance (http://apps.who.int/iris/bitstream/handle/10665/254883/9789241511827-eng.pdf;jsessionid=A02E39F951E42C6E3319FB767C795D2C?sequence=1).

The assessment of health status must include any negative, unwanted, and/or unexpected secondary detrimental effects triggered by the event itself or resulting from an intervention delivered during the event. The post-event findings must be compared to what is known to have existed in the community before the event (pre-event health status). Repeated assessments related to the intervention can be conducted concurrently (in real time) at any point during the event or after the event (during relief and recovery) to determine outcomes of the intervention.

Each intervention must be evaluated in terms of whether the results achieved their objectives in terms of measurable benefits (outcomes), the timeliness and efficiency with which the intervention was delivered, and the associated costs. The continuity in health services is the ultimate goal of any intervention in a disaster, as it encompasses whatever will provide for the overall well-being of the impacted community as a whole (water, shelter, food, etc.)

The primary goal of emergency public health is to prevent or mitigate the deterioration of the physical and mental health status of the disaster-impacted community, in particular its vulnerable populations, such as the chronically ill, elderly, disabled, women, and children, as well as displaced persons (i.e. refugees). Emergency health operations include ensuring access to basic medical and psychological services to survivors, as well as the logistics of prompt restoration of operations at damaged medical facilities (Foege, 1986; Shoaf and Rottman, 2000).

The compartmentalization of the health and medical response into functional units facilitates standardized evaluation. As such, none of the listed components is without influence on public health or human well-being. It is not possible to consider these without thinking of public health. This is exemplified in the health indicators used for assessment of the status of public health activities which are shown in Box 4.2 (Malilay, 2000).

Needs Identification

In the case of a health disaster the identification of the health needs of the injured and the uninjured survivors in the form of emergency care, food, adequate clothing, and shelter is of critical importance and must be met within the shortest time period possible to reduce morbidity and mortality and long-term disability. Major problems in the technical field of needs identification include the development of methods, procedures, and technology to rapidly estimate the total affected population; total number of killed and seriously injured and their locations; number of hospitals destroyed or disabled, as well as those still operating; type and severity of injuries; and types and quantities of medical and surgical services, medical supplies, and pharmaceuticals needed (Smith, 1989; Anker, 1991). It is essential to determine if and when to request assistance from regional and national authorities.

These decisions are critical for lifesaving efforts because time is a risk factor for death and disability. They are usually the responsibility of local authorities (i.e. the mayor, governor, or their designees) and are usually made in conjunction with the incident commander and local health and EMS officials. Delays in initiating or inaccuracy of needs identification is a major cause of delays in the timely delivery of emergency care and, as a result, may lead to

Box 4.2 Suggested indicators for evaluation of quality of public health activities

- Number of out-of-hospital vs. in-hospital deaths
- Hospital admissions per day post impact
- Modes of transport of casualties
- Total number of casualties transported (to local facilities and to outside facilities)
- Number of persons displaced
- Number of shelters deployed to disaster zone
- Pharmaceuticals
  - Availability
  - Sources
  - Distribution
- Food supply
  - Availability
  - Sources
  - Distribution
- Potable water
  - Availability
  - Sources
  - Distribution
- Sanitation (as indicated by number of persons with access to a toilet)

preventable deaths and disabilities, especially among the critically injured. This was a major failure after the 2005 Hurricane Katrina in New Orleans (De Lisi, 2006) and, more recently, after the 2017 Hurricane Maria on the island of Puerto Rico. (https://publichealth.gwu.edu/sites/default/files/downloads/projects/PRstudy/Acertainment%20of%20the%20Estimated%20Excess%20Mortality%20from%20Hurricane%20Maria%20in%20Puerto%20Rico.pdf).

Many disaster experts today consider disaster medicine a sub-discipline of public health. Moreover, many of the minimum standards and indicators defined in the Sphere Project (Sphere Project, 2011) or the Utstein Style Guidelines (Sundnes, 1999) relate to the public health emergency system and its supporting BSFs (basic societal/support functions). As mentioned, evaluation of public health response after a disaster is facilitated by the evaluators' understanding of the level of development and degree of disaster preparedness that existed before the disaster. The identification and selection of well-established descriptive epidemiological health indicators such as case fatality and casualty rates as well as case control studies are essential research tools in the understanding and evaluation of risk and health severity of the event (Binder and Sanderson, 1987; Woodruff et al., 1988; Seaman, 1990; Glass and Noji, 1992; Noji et al., 2000). It also is necessary to choose indicators that accurately capture the scope and quality of health activities during the event. Indices that are useful for the evaluation of the health severity of disaster are listed in Box 4.3.

These data are critical for the evaluation study but reported in isolation will only provide a partial picture of what happened. For these reasons background information collected concurrently or in a systemic fashion from eyewitnesses, and data collected from a review of medical records and autopsy reports, if

Box 4.3 Suggested minimum data set for uniform reporting on the severity of the health disaster

- ◆ Number of affected people as a proportion of total number of people at risk (Total pop. affected/Total pop. at risk)
- ◆ Demographics of casualties (age and gender)
- ◆ Number of injured and killed (crude casualty and mortality rates)
- ◆ Type, mechanism, circumstances and severity of injury/illness, (i.e. crush injury from building collapse, drowning from flooding, acute radiation poisoning from nuclear exposure, asphyxiation from chemical or biological attack, etc.); if possible using standard scoring schemes [Glasgow Coma Scale, injury severity score (ISS), triage category etc.) and ICD-10 codes/E-codes
- ◆ Causes of death
- ◆ Types and location of medical intervention (classified according to ICD procedure codes)
- ◆ Number and location of disabled, partially or fully destroyed medical facilities in the disaster zone, as a proportion of total medical facilities functioning prior to the event (#facilities disabled/Total medical facilities)

    Outcomes (total hospital admissions, excess mortality, other) available, cross-checked with data collected during post disaster field surveys contribute to a more reliable reconstruction of the events that led to injury and death (Ricci et al., 1991).

Disease Surveillance

Epidemiological surveillance aims to establish population-based monitoring systems to prevent, reduce, or track disease outbreaks in in the affected community in the aftermath of a disaster (Surmieda et al., 1992). These epidemiological objectives can be succinctly defined as the surveillance cycle: (1) identification of cases; (2) processing and analysis of data and information; and (3) response to the conclusions. Field surveillance methods vary greatly. Field surveys within the context of the evaluative study must be simple and should address the essential basic questions requiring immediate answers that will inform on the loss of life, illness, or injury. Surveys can address issues such as the availability of medical care, when and how the care was accessed (hospitals, clinics, mobile hospitals, etc.), decontamination and quarantine, and mode of transportation of casualties to medical facilities, and so on (Sundnes and Haimanot, 1993).

Supply Chain Management

Preparedness depends, in part, upon the robustness of community and hospital disaster planning, the amount and types of commodities that were available in stock prior to the disaster, and when and how additional supplies were provided after the event. This may differ from country to country and also within a country. A successful disaster response is defined by early identification of needs, and rapid establishment of a supply chain for each critical need. The evaluation study should focus on the timing and adequacy of delivery and re-supply of manpower, food, shelter, potable water, pharmaceuticals, and medical equipment.

Several countries have contingency legislation that provides standards as to how many days of supplies a health care institution must keep on hand. In some countries, a 60-day supply is required; in other countries, only three days of supplies are required. In still other countries, the amount of supplies required in cache (warehouse facilities) is not regulated; however, the legal directives have proven difficult to enforce. The WHO has developed a hospital emergency response checklist (http://www.euro.who.int/data/assets/pdf_file/0008/268766/Hospital-emergency-response-checklist-Eng.pdf). Consequently, it is not sufficient to assume that the formal requirements of a country are being met. What should be known is what actually is readily available and whether the supplies match the actual needs. Further, it is essential to identify whether contingency plans exist for resupply in the event of a disaster. These considerations apply to back-up emergency lifelines, such as power, food on hand, gas supply, etc. (Kai et al., 1994).

Integrity of Hospital Services

In a disaster the objective is to reduce 'preventable' morbidity and mortality. These are by definition illnesses, injuries, and deaths that would not have occurred under normal emergency conditions. Apart from measures to prevent damage and injury, preventing or reducing morbidity and mortality is crucially dependent on the timeliness and quality of the care provided to seriously injured casualties, both at the scene of injury/illness (field emergency care) and at hospitals that continue to operate as the disaster is unfolding. Determination of the quality and outcome of care is a major objective of the evaluative study. Establishing a consensus on a minimum data set will facilitate uniform data reporting for evaluation and research, enabling the creation of a disaster registry (Box 4.4).

Some of the traditional descriptors of the quality of medical services delivered may not have much relevance in the context of a disaster. For example, merely identifying the number of beds or the number of hospitals per capita would be insufficient. Simply adding a measure of the average distance required for the population to reach an operating medical facility renders the picture more complete; but such information may be so difficult to obtain that to acquire

---

Box 4.4 Suggested critical time points for uniform reporting of medical care activities

- Time of onset/impact
- Time of declaration of disaster situation by government officials
- Time of activation of emergency operations center
- Time first ambulance and/or search and rescue units/medical teams dispatched
- Time of arrival of first responders/medical teams to the disaster zone
- Time of arrival of first casualties to medical facilities
- Time of restoration of hospital services in disabled/damaged facilities
- Time of restoration of full hospital services
- Time of restoration of lifelines to hospital facilities

it may be counter-productive. Therefore, the number of hospitals per defined size of a geographic area may be adequate, but this number may not address all of the details noted above. Several types of information may have limited value, depending on what is being studied. The number of inhabitants per physician is an indicator of the availability of higher levels of medical care. A large number does not necessarily mean that health care has been neglected as non-physicians may provide much of the basic health care. The number of inhabitants per health worker (licensed) may help to complete the picture. A high number of health workers in a population, relative to the number of physicians, may indicate that primary health care has been given priority in order to meet the most basic health and public health needs of the population at large.

Further, the top five diseases treated before the disaster in the hospitals in the affected region is an important indicator, not only of which problems require ongoing medical treatment, but also what were the usual types of medical care at a given hospital or clinic, or was the medical facility adaptable to emergency conditions. Thus, many of the questions asked in an evaluative study seek an answer comprised not only of a number, but also qualitative descriptions. The primary, secondary, and tertiary levels of medical care may have a different meaning in an urban industrialized area (Aoki et al, 2004) compared to a rural area in a developing country (Haiti, Bangladesh). However, both scenarios may have medical care levels based on primary health care, a district hospital(s), county hospital(s), and a central hospital. Without an interview-based description, these differences may be missed, and incorrect assumptions may result. Such important differences may not be detected from the use of surveys and can only partly be quantified.

The limitations associated with the quantification of emergency medical services (EMS) systems are similar. A proper description of the EMS system requires more than quantitative indicators such as the number and type of vehicles normally used to provide these services, or numbers and levels of training of emergency responders. The type of training provided and to whom it is provided, the density of calls, mechanisms of finance, response times, means of transport, etc., all constitute information necessary to get a valid picture of the technical capacities and of other capabilities or limitations of such services. However qualitative assessment of how these assets were organized and managed, and barriers which may have occurred to prevent their implementation under disaster conditions, is essential for a full understanding of the response effort.

Failure of the medical system can occur in the delivery of primary, secondary, tertiary, and/or critical care services. In sudden-onset disasters, the most common early inadequacies occur in the delivery of prehospital emergency care. During such events, this function is typically linked closely with the Search and Rescue function, particularly during the out-of-hospital phase. The degree of failure of pre-hospital and in-hospital EMS must be measured against the level of such services available during the pre-event phase.

Ideally, the emergency medical care function is initiated by first responders, followed by emergency medical and surgical treatment to *individual* patients in the field and definitive care in hospitals. The standard of care differs from the emergency response that is possible during everyday emergencies. However, the key functions within the EMS/trauma domain that should be at the center of the evaluative study include, but are not limited to, urban search and rescue, the process of triage and diagnoses, prehospital treatment, evacuation, and transportation of casualties out of the disaster zone to medical facilities. These activities encompass primary, secondary, and tertiary care. Time is a critical risk factor for injury and death in disaster, and as such should be evaluated as an indicator of quality of the care delivered (Box 4.4).

Mass Casualty Management

Search and rescue is the process of detecting, identifying, extricating, and gathering or collecting victims from the scene of injury or illness (e.g. extrication from under rubble). It may also include transport to nearby staging areas or casualty collection points (CCP) within the tactical area of operations, where further harm is avoided and from which patients are initially administered prehospital treatment, prepared for transport, and loaded onto emergency transport vehicles. In the case of chemical release or exposure to biological agents, patients are decontaminated in pre-designated areas by properly trained emergency responders equipped with the proper personal protective gear, prior to transportation to a treatment facility or placed in isolation units, thus protecting rescuers and other individuals from lethal exposure.

Once casualties are rescued, cleared from the immediate disaster area, and transported to a casualty collection point or a medical facility, triage and initial treatment are performed. Triage is the method by which the type, extent, and severity of injury or illness sustained by a disaster victim is prioritized for treatment (Perelmut and Pretto, 2019). While the severity of illness is typically the most important factor in the prioritization of standard medical care, the goal of care during a mass casualty incident is to maximize overall patient survival. In order to accomplish this goal critically ill or moribund victims are often given lower priority than less critical patients who are more likely to survive with treatment. Triage should be carried-out by physicians with advanced trauma life support (ATLS) training familiar with triage methods (Table 4.1).

Table 4.1 Triage categories

Category	Implicated actions	Characteristics
T1–IMMEDIATE	Immediate life-saving interventions and immediate evacuation	Patients with life-threatening injuries but a high chance of survival when treated
T2–URGENT	Initial treatment Reassessment Rapid evacuation	Patients with severe injuries but not in immediate critical condition
T3–DELAYED	First aid supplies Reassessment Transport	Patient with minor injuries able to care for themselves
DEAD	Transport	Patients declared dead by a medical professional or with non-survivable injuries and no vital signs
T4–EXPECTANT	Supportive pain control and anxiolytic treatment only Reassessment Transport	Patients with serious injuries expected to die Only to be used when authorized by declaration of a mass casualty situation

In a disaster, mass casualty management requires a series of interventions that are quantitatively and qualitatively different from the everyday emergency situation or multi-casualty incident (MCI), such as a bus or train accident, which by definition does not overwhelm the local EMS/trauma care system. Ideally, these disaster medical management functions are most effective for lifesaving when they are implemented in a timely manner by well-organized, experienced EMS/trauma services systems consisting of trained bystanders (e.g. community emergency response teams, first responders, ground and air ambulance EMT/paramedic units; trauma teams/hospitals, and network of community hospitals pre-existing in the community. However, it is important to note that the standard of care in mass casualty and catastrophic disaster events will differ markedly from everyday EMS/trauma care. According to NATO guidelines, bystander response within 10 minutes, 1 hour to achieve transport to a treatment facility, and 2 hours to definitive care or damage control surgery (Committee of Chiefs of the Military Medical Services, NATO 2015). During this time frame, however, 'preventable' deaths may occur that would not have occurred under 'normal' conditions.

Emergency medical services (EMS) systems provide medical treatment to ill or injured patients. The *medical* system provides for the identification of casualties, assessment of symptoms and signs, triage, and the transport of casualties for definitive diagnosis and treatment of patients. It includes primary, secondary, and tertiary care when appropriate in the field or in hospitals (Figure 4.3).

The quality of EMS systems varies extensively from region to region within a country and also from country to country. In some cases there are wide variations in capacity between neighboring districts within a country. When assessing medical care, therefore, it is mandatory that the level and the nature of the care that was available prior to the disaster be identified.

In major disasters casualties are usually not transported in ambulances (Angus et al., 1991, 1997; Abrams et al., 1991; Pretto et al., 1992, 1994; Bissell et al., 1994). Instead, uninjured or lightly injured co-victims carry out this function using whatever means is available for transport (private care, bus, train, wagon, etc.). Bystanders are usually the relatives, friends, or neighbors of the injured (Abrams et al., 1991). Once professional rescuers and emergency medical personnel initiate their operations, transport of critically injured casualties is done by land or air ambulance (helicopters) from casualty collection points close to the disaster zone to treatment facilities outside the tactical area of operations; whenever possible, and especially when extended transport times are anticipated, casualties should be accompanied by health care professionals with, at minimum, advanced trauma or cardiac life support expertise if available. The lack of ambulances, helicopters, and so on, and traffic jams or disruption of roads and highways to and from the disaster area due to destruction or debris are frequent causes of delay in the transport of casualties.

Pre-hospital Treatment

Field medical care is the spectrum of triage and lifesaving interventions applied in the pre-hospital setting by bystanders, first responders, and emergency medical personnel on casualties of disaster (Garner et al., 2001; Iserson and Moskop, 2007; Perelmut and Pretto, 2019). The objective is to apply first aid and control life-threatening bleeding or compromised airway prior to transport. Usually, field medical care, especially 'resuscitative surgery' or 'damage control surgery' is performed only when the type and severity of illness or injury threaten life or limb, precluding safe transport to a treatment facility. In general, there are five main types of field medical care or damage control interventions (Perelmut and Pretto , 2019):

1) *Life-supporting first aid (LSFA):* Involves the delivery of basic first aid by trained uninjured survivors or co-victims and is aimed at initiating the life support chain. Box 4.5 describes recommended bystander life supporting first aid (LSFA) maneuvers (Pretto et al., 1991; Pretto, 2018).

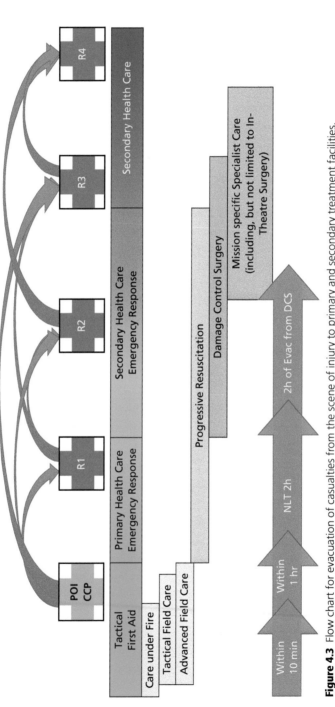

Figure 4.3 Flow chart for evacuation of casualties from the scene of injury to primary and secondary treatment facilities.
Reproduced from *Allied Joint Publication For Medical Support (AJP) 4.10.* © NATO/OTAN, 2015.

> # Box 4.5 Guidelines for bystander life supporting first aid (LSFA) response in disasters
>
> - Calling for help
> - Knowing when to approach a victim in a hazardous environment
> - Maintaining a patent airway in an unconscious but breathing patient (i.e., triple airway maneuver)
> - External hemorrhage control
> - Positioning for shock
> - Rescue pull (removing the victim from imminent danger)
> - CPR (rarely indicated in a disaster).

2) *Basic rescue or extrication:* In situations involving collapsed structures it involves the simple extrication of victims from vehicles or those buried under light rubble. It is usually performed by uninjured co-victims within the immediate disaster zone equipped only with bare hands, minimal supplies, or improvised tools. However, there are some basic techniques that can be learned by the public at large (Abrams et al., 1991).

3) *Basic trauma life support (BTLS):* Constitutes the second step in the life support chain involving the application of advanced first aid techniques, such as the following: airway control with or without adjuncts, external hemorrhage control, immobilization of unstable limb fractures, placement of peripheral intravenous lines, wound dressing, initial burn treatment, and other lifesaving maneuvers by trained first responders.

4) *Advanced trauma life support (ATLS):* The application of triage and lifesaving emergency medical or surgical treatment to critically injured patients by physicians (Box 4.6).

5) *Resuscitative surgery:* This type of surgery involves circumscribed surgical procedures performed in the field with general or regional anesthesia to prevent loss of life or limb due to external or internal abdominal, thoracic or cerebral hemorrhage or prevention of wound infection (gangrene), compartment syndrome, etc. (Box 4.7).

Hospital Treatment

Hospital response during a disaster is driven by the hospital's external disaster response plan, whose organization should incorporate the incident management system as modified for hospital operations.

Box 4.6 Advanced trauma life support maneuvers and interventions

- Definitive airway management with endotracheal intubation, if necessary
- Assisted ventilation
- Establishing Intravenous access
- Central venous line placement for volume resuscitation
- Administration of vasoactive medication and antidotes as needed
- Chest tube placement (pneumothorax; hemothorax)
- Wound packing

Casualties evacuated to hospitals for definitive care, which is defined as the delivery of specialized corrective medical or surgical treatment in a field hospital or permanent medical facility. These interventions are carried out by physicians, surgeons, nurses, and other health care professionals. The objectives are stabilization of vital signs, reversal of life-threatening illness or injury, and the prevention of long-term disability or death.

In the United States, the Joint Commission for Accreditation of Health Care Organizations (JCAHO) provides direction but limited detail regarding

Box 4.7 Damage control resuscitation

- Volume resuscitation (fluid and blood component administration) to prevent shock (NB: permissive hypotension)
- Emergency exploratory surgery with general and/or regional anesthesia techniques:
  - laparotomy
  - thoracotomy
  - craniotomy
- Wound debridement
- Limb amputation performed in the out-of-hospital setting usually to prevent loss of life due to, gangrene, compartment syndrome, etc. (Missair, 2010)

Box 4.8 Checklist for evaluation of hospital disaster preparedness

- A plan for the acquisition and deployment of necessary medical equipment, supplies, and pharmaceuticals.
- A plan for emergency backup lifeline (power, gas, water, food) and personnel recall (medical and nonmedical) to allow continuous operations for, at minimum, 24-72 hours.
- Hospital staff services were reorganized for disaster operations by recalling and reassigning personnel to deal promptly and effectively with a surge of casualties (casualty estimates and surge capacity needs to be determined beforehand).
- Mutual aid and liaison agreements with neighboring hospitals/EMS systems were activated and implemented.
- Local communication network with prehospital EMS ambulance units, other hospitals in the network, local and state health authorities, families of casualties, the media, and the emission of periodic updates or situation reports.
- Surge capacity plan (see next section for a full description)
- Transport plan for the transfer/discharge of stable inpatients or diversion of disaster casualties to other health care institutions, nursing homes, outpatient facilities, home, and so on.
- Documentation of admission and care provided to casualties by hospital personnel that is independent of power supply.
- Inpatient tracking, both before and after admission.
- Designation of triage and treatment areas within the hospital with prioritization of care.

hospital disaster plans or hospital disaster management functions. However, the hospital incident management system has been developed to organize hospital disaster response activities around a set of specific and measurable objectives that define the hospital's performance in the event of a disaster (Ricci and Pretto, 1991). Box 4.8 lists disaster preparedness and response activities in the hospital setting during disaster (Box 4.9).

Surge capacity: Hospital external disaster response plans often lack an important component of a hospital's response to a disaster, namely the

Box 4.9 Checklist for evaluation of hospital disaster/emergency management

- Leadership and management team based on the hospital incident management system to lead and coordinate the hospital's response.
- Casualty reception and triage areas (usually the emergency room and adjacent areas), with patients segregated according to their need for treatment but also according to infectious disease status or chemical or radiological contaminated.
- Decontamination/isolation areas (in the event of casualties of chemical, biological, radiological attack or pandemic influenza)
- Designated areas for the diagnosis, treatment, or stabilization of patients who have life-threatening conditions (RED) such as acute respiratory failure, who require intensive care for immediate and continuous physiologic monitoring, medical or surgical intervention, and or mechanical ventilation
- Designated area for the diagnosis, treatment, or stabilization of patients having urgent conditions (YELLOW) who will be referred for follow-up care
- Designated area for the treatment of patients with non-urgent conditions (GREEN), with referral for later definitive diagnosis, treatment, and comprehensive care
- Designated area for the reception of moribund or dead casualties (GRAY/BLACK) or for pain management and pastoral services.
- Selection of alternate treatment areas (outside the hospital) in the event the hospital must be evacuated or cannot provide services. In some situations hospital personnel may be compelled to evacuate the facility and to deliver medical and surgical services in the out-of-hospital setting, severely hampering the hospital's ability to function.

incorporation of a critical care expansion plan to ensure surge capacity. Critical care surge capacity can be defined as the maximal number of patients that can receive adequate critical care for as long as required, after recruiting all critical care resources (Perelmut and Pretto, 2019).

When assessing a surge capacity plan, it is important to review services delivered. For example, did pharmacy, laboratory, radiology, respiratory therapy, and nutritional services provide adequate services during the disaster? Did stockpiling of resources including equipment, supplies, and pharmaceuticals prior to the disaster meet the needs of the surge in casualties? Ventilators are often limited in a surge capacity scenario and hospitals working alone are unlikely to be able to provide enough ventilators to support the critically ill. A regional count of ventilators should be performed, with multiple hospitals working together to create a mass disaster 'critical care' operational plan (The ANZIC Influenza Investigators, 2009).

Delivery of critical care during a disaster or pandemic not only depends on the allocation of appropriate physical resources, but hospitals must ensure sufficient numbers of trained medical, nursing, and ancillary staff (Nap et al., 2008; Missair et al., 2010, Missair et al., 2013). A disaster response is likely to consume the available reserves of rested personnel within 24–48 hours, and hospitals should use adaptive measures to provide appropriate staffing in these scenarios, such as shorter shifts (i.e. 4–6 hours) to avoid fatigue and exhaustion. While the standard nurse to patient ratio in North American ICUs is 1:1 or 1:2, this isn't practical during a critical care surge. Strategies used to mitigate the potential for patient harm due to this change in ratio include creation of nursing care teams, with the use of non-critical care nurses to perform tasks within their skill sets in order to off-load the demands of the ICU nurses.

Mass Fatality Management (Mortuary Services)

A critical function within the public health domain is the establishment of the infrastructure for the safe and correct transport and disposition of fatalities (Hooft et al., 1989). Depending on local cultural and religious norms this may require the identification and establishment of decontamination and disposal/burial areas at a distance from the disaster zone. Failure to adequately perform this function may lead to disease outbreaks or wider spread of infectious diseases, as was observed during the Ebola epidemic of Western Africa in 2013. However, 'unsolicited' mass burials are mostly incorrect and unnecessary and create other challenges to society (de Ville de Goyet, 1999).

Summary

In this chapter we have presented the major components of a generalized medical and public health disaster response system. These components will be employed in Part 2 of this Field Manual to construct the sample logic model and minimum data set presented in Chapters 7 and 8.

References

Abrams, J.I., Pretto, E., Angus, D., and Safar, P. (1991). Basic Extrication Training of the Lay Public for Disaster Preparedness. *Prehospital and Disaster Medicine*. **6**, pp. 547.

Angus, D., Pretto, E., Abrams, J.I., et al. (1997). Epidemiologic Assessment of Building Collapse Pattern, Mortality, and Medical Response After the 1992 Earthquake in Erzincan, Turkey. *Prehospital and Disaster Medicine*. **12** (3), pp. 222–231.

Angus, D., Pretto, E., Abrams, J.I., and Safar, P. (1991). Life Supporting First Aid Training of the Lay Public for Disaster Preparedness. *Prehospital and Disaster Medicine*. **6**, pp. 547.

Anker, M. (1991). Epidemiological and Statistical Methods for Rapid Health Assessment: Introduction. *World Health Statistics Quarterly*. **44**, pp. 94–97.

Aoki, N., Nishimura N., Pretto, E., et. al. (2004). Survival and Cost Analysis of Fatalities of the Kobe Earthquake in Japan. *Prehospital Emergency Care*. **8**, pp. 217–222.

Binder, S. and Sanderson, L.M. (1987). The Role of Epidemiologist in Natural Disasters. *Annals of Emergency Medicine*. **16**, pp. 1081–1084.

Bissell, R., Pretto, E., Angus, D., et al. (1994). Post-Preparedness Disaster Response in Costa Rica. *Prehospital and Disaster Medicine*. **9** (2), pp. 96–106.

Chan, T.C., Killeen, J., Griswold, W., and Lenert, L. (2004). Information Technology and Emergency Medical Care During Disasters. *Academic Emergency Medicine*. **11** (11), pp. 1229–1236.

Committee of the Chiefs of Military Medical Service, Allied Joint Publication 4.10: 2015, Allied Joint Doctrine for Medical Support, NATO Standardization Agreements.

De Lisi, L.E. (2006). The Katrina Disaster and Its Lessons. *World Psychiatry*. **5** (1), pp. 3–4.

Federal Emergency Management System. NRF resource center. Available at: http://www.fema.gov/emergency/nrf/. Accessed on: July 22, 2010.

Foege, W.H. (1986). Public health aspects of disaster management. In: Last, J.M, ed., *Public Health and Preventive Medicine*, 1st ed. Norwalk: Appleton-Century-Crofts.

Garner, A., Lee, A., Harrison, K., and Schultz, C.H. (2001). Comparative Analysis of Multiple Casualty Incident Triage Algorithms. *Annals of Emergency Medicine*. **38**, pp. 541–548.

Glass, R.I. and Noji, E.K. (1992). Epidemiologic surveillance following disasters. In: Halperin, W.E., Baker, E.L., and Monson, R.R., eds. *Public Health Surveillance*, 1st ed. New York: Van Nostrand, Reinhold.

WHO. (1970). *Health Aspects of Chemical and Biological Weapons*. Report of WHO Group Consultants. Geneva, Switzerland: World Health Organization.

Hooft, P.J., Noji, E.K., and Van de Voorde, H.P. (1989). Fatality Management in Mass-Casualty Incidents. *Forensic Science International*. **40**, pp. 3–14.

Iserson, K.V. and Moskop, J.C. (2007). Triage in Medicine, Part I: Concept, History, and Types. *Annals of Emergency Medicine*. **49** (3), pp. 275–281.

Kai T, Ukai K, Ohta M., and Pretto, E. (1994). Hospital disaster preparedness in Osaka, Japan. *Prehospital and Disaster Medicine*. **9** (1), pp. 29–34.

Malilay, J. (2000). Public Health Assessments in Disaster Settings: Recommendations for a Multidisciplinary Approach. *Prehospital and Disaster Medicine*. **15** (4), pp. 167–172.

Missair, A., Gebhard, R., Pierre, E., et al. (2010). Surgical Care Amid the Rubble During the January 12, 2010 Earthquake in Haiti: The Importance of Regional Anesthesia. Prehospital and Disaster Medicine 2010 Nov-Dec;25(6) pp. 487-93

Missair, A. Pretto E.A., Visan A., et al (2013) Lobo, L. A matter of life or limb? A review of traumatic injury patterns and anesthesia techniques for disaster relief in major earthquakes. Anesth Analg. 2013, Oct 117(4) pp. 934-1

Molino, L.N. (2006). *Emergency Incident Management Systems: Fundamentals and Applications*. Hoboken, NJ: John Wiley and Sons, p. 518.

Nap, R.E., Andriessen, M., Meesen, N.E.L., et al. (2008). Pandemic Influenza and Excess Intensive Care Workload. *Emerging Infectious Diseases*. **14** (10), pp. 1518–1525.

Noji, E.K. (2000). The Public Health Consequences of Disasters. *Prehospital Disaster Medicine*. **15** (4), pp. 147–157.

Perelmut, R. and Pretto E. (2019) Anesthetic considerations in homeland disasters. In: Urman R, Gross WL, Phillips B., eds., *Anesthesia Outside of the Operating Room*. Oxford, UK: Oxford University Press, pp. 384

Pretto, E., Angus, D., Abrams, J.I., et al. (1994). An Analysis of Prehospital Mortality in an Earthquake. *Prehospital Disaster Medicine*. **9** (2), pp. 107–117.

Pretto, E., Ricci, E., Safar, P., et al. (1992). Disaster Reanimatology Potentials: A Structured Interview Study in Armenia III: Results, Conclusions, and Recommendations. *Prehospital Disaster Medicine*. **7** (4), pp. 327–338.

Ricci, E. and Pretto, E. (1991). Assessment of Prehospital and Hospital Response in Disaster. *Critical Care Clinics*. **7** (2), pp. 471–484.

Ricci, E., Pretto, E., Safar, P., et al. (1991). Disaster Reanimatology Potentials: A Structured Interview Study in Armenia II. Method for the Evaluation of Medical Response to Major Disasters. *Prehospital Disaster Medicine*. **6** (2), pp. 159–166.

Rubinson, L. and O'Toole, T. (2005). Critical Care During Epidemics. *Critical Care*. **9**, pp. 311–313.

Seaman, J. (1990). Disaster Epidemiology: Or Why Most International Disaster Relief is Ineffective. *Injury*. **21**, pp. 5–8.

Shoaf, K.I. and Rottman, S.J. (2000). The Role of Public Health in Disaster Medicine. *Prehospital Disaster Medicine*. **15** (4), pp. 145–213.

Smith, G.S. (1989). Development of Rapid Epidemiologic Assessment Methods to Evaluate Health Status and Delivery of Health Services. *International Journal of Epidemiology*. **18**, S2–S15.

Stambler, K. and Barbera, J. (2011). Engineering the Incident Command and Multiagency Coordination Systems. *Journal of Homeland Security and Emergency Management*. **8** (1), pp. 1547–7355.

Sundnes K.O. (1999). Health disaster management: guidelines for evaluation and research in the Utstein Style: executive summary. Task force for quality control of disaster management. Prehosp and Disaster Med. Apr.-June 14(2) pp. 42-53.

Sundnes, K.O.,(ed.). (2014). Operational Framework. *Scandinavian Journal of Public Health*. **42** (14), pp. 83.

Sundnes, K.O. and Haimanot, A.T. (1993). Epidemic of Louse-borne Relapsing Fever in Ethopia. *Lancet*, **342**, pp. 1213–1215.

Surmieda, M.R.S., Abad-Viola, G., Abellanosa, I.P., et al. (1992). Surveillance in Evacuation Camps After the Eruption of Mt. Pinatubo. *Morbidity and Mortality Weekly Report: Surveillance Summaries*. **41** (4), pp. 9–12.

The ANZIC Influenza Investigators. (2009). Critical Care Services and 2009 H1N1 Influenza in Australia and New Zealand. *New England Journal of Medicine*. **361**, pp. 1925–1934.

Ville de Goyet, C. (1999). Stop Propagating Disaster Myths. AUJIEmMGMT 55; 14(4).

Woodruff, B., Toole, J.M., and Rodriguez, D.C., et al. (1990). Disease Surveillance and Control After a Flood in Khartoum, Sudan, 1988. *Disasters*. **14**, pp. 151–163.

Part 2

How to Design and Implement a Disaster Evaluation Study

An Eight-step Approach

In Part 2, we describe an *eight-step approach* to the conduct of a comprehensive scientific evaluation of the medical and public health response to disasters. While the authors of this Field Manual understand that time and resource constraints can prevent the full application of each step in our suggested model for each disaster, we strongly encourage evaluation teams to address and include, to the extent possible, each step when designing and implementing future evaluation studies. However, each step may be expanded or shortened consistent with the time and resources that are available for the evaluation study. Also certain steps may be carried out concurrently. The recommended steps in the eight-step model are: (1) evaluation team leader identifies stakeholder group members and calls initial meeting; (2) identify the evaluation questions using categories of evaluation; (3) construct a logic model and research design; (4) prepare 'mixed-methods' data collection instruments; (5) construct a sampling plan; (6) conduct a 'scout survey'; (7) identify and train data collection team members and collect data; and (8) analyze data and prepare a final report.

Graphic Showing 8-Step Approach to Disaster Evaluation

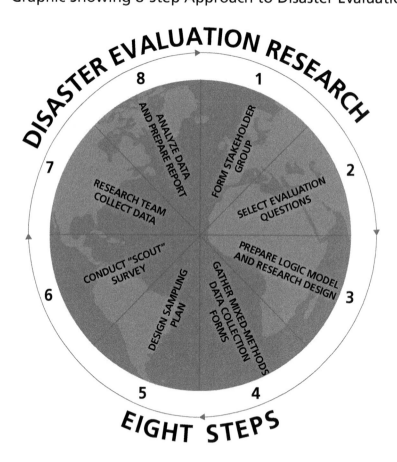

DISASTER EVALUATION RESEARCH

EIGHT STEPS

8 ANALYZE DATA AND PREPARE REPORT

1 FORM STAKEHOLDER GROUP

2 SELECT EVALUATION QUESTIONS

3 PREPARE LOGIC MODEL AND RESEARCH DESIGN

GATHER MIXED-METHODS DATA COLLECTION FORMS

4

DESIGN SAMPLING PLAN

5

CONDUCT "SCOUT" SURVEY

6

RESEARCH TEAM COLLECT DATA

7

Chapter 5

Form the Stakeholder Group (Step 1)

Keypoints

If an evaluation study is ultimately to be used to change and improve the medical and public health response to disasters it is essential to involve those who have the strongest interest and reasons for making improvements and who have the power and resources to do so. These individuals are referred to as 'stakeholders'. Experience has shown clearly that if the key stakeholders are involved from the beginning in the planning and implementation of the evaluation, and in the process of preparing recommendations for change in future preparedness and response efforts, the evaluation recommendations are much more likely to be adopted. The evaluation team leader, after review of source material such as governmental reports, organization charts, newspaper and agency descriptions, should select appropriate members of the group.

The Initiation of an Evaluation Study

The first step in planning an evaluation study of the medical and public health response to a disaster is to identify the key 'stakeholders'. This is best accomplished by the designated Evaluation Team Leader after he/she reviews information about the response effort. This information may include government agency reports, newspaper accounts, tables of organization for organizations that participated in the preparedness and relief effort, as well reports prepared by participating non-governmental organizations. Stakeholders are individuals who, for various reasons, have a deep interest in the results of the evaluation study and who have sufficient influence to bring about any recommended changes that might emerge from the evaluation.

One of the most important distinguishing features of evaluation studies is that they are inherently political in nature. Carol Weiss, one of the first university-based evaluation methodologists, put the issue succinctly:

> Knowing that political constraints and resistances exist is not a reason for abandoning evaluation research; rather it is a precondition for useable evaluation research. Only when the evaluator has insights into interests and motivations of other actors in the system, into the roles that he/she is consciously or inadvertently playing, the obstacles that impinge upon the evaluation effort, and the limitations and possibilities for putting evaluation to work, – only with sensitivity to the politics of evaluation research – can the evaluator be as creative and useful as he/she should be.
>
> (Weiss, 1993)

In the same article, Weiss identified three ways in which politics and evaluation are intertwined.

> First, programs and policies are 'creatures of political decisions' so evaluations implicitly judge those decisions. Secondly, evaluations feed political decision making and compete with other perspectives in the political process. Finally, evaluation is political by its very nature because of the issues it addresses and the conclusions it reaches.
>
> (Weiss, 1993)

The analysis of the political dimension of evaluation studies by Weiss and others was an important breakthrough in the development of evaluation science. It is safe to say that the very first evaluators had rather utopian and perhaps naive ideas about evaluation in that they assumed that the 'facts' about the effectiveness (or not) of a program or intervention would be accepted at face value and then used to inform policy setting and program change. As noted by Weiss in describing the optimism held by many in the academic and political worlds that societal ills could be remedied if programs were based in science and then scientifically evaluated:

> There was much hoopla about the rationality that social science would bring to the untidy world of government. It would provide hard data for planning ... and give cause and effect theories for policy making, so that statesmen would know which variables to alter in order to effect the desired outcomes .... And once policies were in operation, it would provide objective valuation of their effectiveness so that necessary modifications could be made to improve performance.
>
> (Weiss, 1977)

This expectation proved to be quite naïve because human nature, and the world of rewards and punishments in which we live and work, causes most of us to avoid negative criticism is spite of its value for improving our own performance and that of programs for which we are responsible. When this awareness of the inherent sensitivity of evaluation findings, and the resultant barrier this imposed to the conduct and ultimate use of evaluation findings became clear, a revised approach to evaluation emerged. The approach is known by several names, but the basic ideas as developed and elaborated upon by Michael Quinn Patton are the most widely followed. In his book, *Utilization Focused Evaluation*, Patton provides a cogent analysis of the problem of the widespread underutilization and politicization of evaluation findings and concludes that the best way to increase utilization is to involve key stakeholders in the evaluation process. In his words:

> Utilization-Focused Evaluation begins with the premise that evaluations should be judged by their utility and actual use; therefore evaluators should … design any evaluation with careful consideration of how everything that is done, from beginning to end, will affect use. … In any evaluation, there are many potential stakeholders and an array of possible uses. Utilization-Focused evaluation requires moving to … actual primary intended users and their explicit commitments to concrete specific uses. The evaluator facilitates judgement and decision making by intended users rather than acting as an … independent judge.
>
> (Patton, 1997)

The importance of Patton's insights and approach cannot be overstated. If the intent is to have the evaluation results used to improve disaster response and preparedness, those individuals who are able to act upon the findings and recommendations should be involved in the evaluation study from beginning to end.

Suggestions for Identifying the Stakeholder Group

We suggest that the stakeholder group contain approximately one or two individuals from each of the four general categories identified below (the 4Ps). We believe that a group of four to eight members would provide adequate direction and buy-in without being unwieldy. The members may be chosen from among the following:

- *Professionals*: Chief Public Health Official; Hospital administrator; Director of Emergency response system; Member of First Responder group; Physician who participated in the rescue operation.
- *Payers*: Representatives of any agency or organization that provided funds or other resources for the preparedness, response and rehabilitation functions: insurance companies, non-governmental organizations, governmental agency that provided funds for preparedness and rescue.
- *Politicians*: Mayor (or Designee) and representative of local governing council.
- *Public*: Victims, relatives of victims, uninjured residents of the disaster area.

Structure and Operation of the Stakeholder Group

The group should be created and convened by the individual selected to lead the evaluation effort (Evaluation Team Leader) in consultation with a public official in the disaster zone. The evaluation team leader should ask for a commitment from each stakeholder to attend three meetings with each meeting to last approximately 2 hours. One member of the stakeholder group should be selected to serve as the Chair.

Meeting 1: The first meeting should be used to reach agreement on the evaluation objectives, questions, and data collection methods and to identify any serious barriers, political or technical, to the conduct of the evaluation. The identified barriers should be discussed and ways to overcome them should be identified.

Meeting 2: The second meeting should be held when the evaluation team returns from the data collection field work, and has prepared a preliminary set of findings and recommendations for stakeholder review and comment. Stakeholders should be encouraged to discuss the conclusions reached and to add or delete any recommendation in the draft report.

Meeting 3: The final meeting of the stakeholder group should be held to review the final draft of the evaluation report, but focusing on the recommendations for improved preparedness and response. If there is a subgroup that disagrees with the recommendations, wholly or in part, they should be asked by the Evaluation Team Leader to prepare a 'minority report' which should be included in the final document.

Desired Characteristics of Stakeholder Groups

The individuals selected for membership in the stakeholder group should have several characteristics.

In general, they should:

- Be in positions of sufficient power and influence that they will be able to influence future preparedness and response decisions.
- Believe the evaluation is important to conduct and be committed to implementing the recommendations.
- Be willing to make a firm commitment of time to attend the meetings of the group.
- Be able to represent and articulate their unique perspective on the events that occurred prior to and during the disaster event.

The above suggestions are based upon the work of Patton (1997).

Summary

We consider the involvement of a carefully selected group of stakeholders, who are knowledgeable and empowered, to be an essential component of any scientific evaluation. If properly selected and involved, this structural component of the evaluation effort should provide a strong impetus toward the implementation of the recommendations contained in the final report. In addition, the stakeholder group will serve as a type of validation of the accuracy of the findings, and they can suggest ways to align recommendations with the cultural context within which they will be expected to be implemented.

Acknowledgment

The extract from Weiss, C., Research for Policy's Sake: The Enlightenment Function of Social Research. *Policy Analyses*. 3 (4), pp. 553–565. Copyright © 1993, Sage Publications, is reproduced here with permission. The extract from Weiss, C., *Using Social Research in Public Policy Making*. Copyright © 1977, Lexington Books, is reproduced here with permission.

References

Patton, M.Q. (1997). *Utilization Focused Evaluation*, 3rd ed. Thousand Oaks, CA: Sage Publications, p. 20.

Weiss, C. (ed.) (1977). *Using Social Research in Public Policy Making*. Lexington, MA: Lexington Books, p. 4.

Weiss, C. (1977). Research for Policy's Sake; The Enlightenment Function of Social Research. *Policy Analyses*. 3 (4), pp. 553–565.

Weiss, C. (1993). Where Politics and Evaluation Meet. *Evaluation Practice*. 14 (1), p. 94.

Further reading

Patton, M.Q. (2008). *Utilization Focused Evaluation*, 4th ed. Thousand Oaks, CA: Sage.

Chapter 6

Formulate Evaluation Questions (Step 2)

Keypoints

In this chapter we define the five basic categories of evaluation, namely structure (resources), process (activities), outcomes, adequacy, and costs associated with the response(s). Structure refers to the equipment and personnel and the way in which these resources were organized for use in the medical response. Process refers to the activities carried out during the disaster response. Outcome assessment concerns the results of the care provided on the patients served, usually measured over time. Adequacy describes the extent to which the search-and-rescue, pre-hospital and hospital, and public health responses were able to meet the needs of the community during the disaster response. In general, these categories are consistent with the design of a typical logic model. Following the discussion of 'evaluation categories' we suggest questions that the evaluation team might consider for inclusion in the evaluation study. For each category we suggest questions which could be addressed in any disaster evaluation study which focuses on the medical and public health response. The stakeholder group should be fully involved in the selection of questions to be addressed by the evaluation team.

Five Evaluation Categories

As a way of organizing stakeholder thinking about what overall questions should be addressed by the evaluation study, it is useful to draw upon the major components of a logic model. Evaluators can focus their efforts upon one or more of five basic categories of information. Think of these as separate 'windows' to the reality of the medical and public health response to disasters. That is, each category defines and directs us to examine an important aspect of a large mass of human activity that occurs before, during, and after a disaster. These categories, in general, correspond to the major categories in a logic model. The discussion of categories of evaluation is based upon the work of Suchman (1967) and Ricci and Pretto (1991).

The categories most commonly used in scientific evaluation studies (although not all are addressed in every study) are discussed.

Structure (available resources or inputs) for the Disaster Response

How the medical and public health response is organized, the resources required including equipment and personnel.

Process (activities) Followed in Carrying out the Response

What response activities were actually carried out? How well did the medical and public health components function? How well were individuals prepared? What barriers were encountered and how were these dealt with? Or, were key barriers not overcome? If not, why?

Outcomes (effects of activities) That Were Achieved (or not)

It is useful to think in terms of a progression of outcomes from 'short term–intermediate–long term'. What was and/or was not achieved as a result of the medical and public health response in the short, intermediate, and long term? To what extent were the desired outcomes (e.g. prevention of morbidity and mortality) achieved?

Adequacy of the Disaster Response

As defined by many evaluation scientists, 'adequacy' refers to the extent of death and disability that could have theoretically been prevented (total need) compared with what was actually achieved.

Costs of the Response

What did the medical and public health response cost? Was the money spent most effectively relative to the benefits received? This category, although useful, has not been routinely included in disaster evaluation studies. Hopefully, in the future it will be addressed.

Each of the general questions suggested for the five evaluation categories could be linked to sub-questions. The following are examples of evaluative questions that can be used for each category of evaluation. These are offered only as suggestions for consideration by the stakeholder group and evaluation team. Each evaluation team, working with the stakeholder group, should select the questions in which they are most interested while considering the time and resources (funding) available to conduct the evaluation.

Suggested Questions

Following the reasoning inherent in a logic model, there are three fundamental questions which should be addressed by each Stakeholder Group/Evaluation Team in every disaster evaluation study. They are:

1) Were the resources needed for an effective response available? (If not, what were the deficiencies?) These questions address the category of 'structure' (inputs).

2) Were the response activities implemented as planned? (If not, what barriers were encountered during the implementation process?) These questions address the category of activities.

3) What was the resulting impact of the disaster, and the response, on disaster related morbidity and mortality? These questions address the category of 'outcomes'.

A fourth question is often of interest:

4) What did the response effort cost?

The following specific questions are offered for consideration by each evaluation team/stakeholder group as they plan a disaster evaluation study.

Structure (inputs/resources)

Evaluation of structure could address questions such as:

♦ Were ambulances, hospital emergency department, and critical care units sufficiently equipped and supplied to meet the demands of the disaster?

♦ Were sufficient numbers of properly trained individuals available and properly engaged—especially volunteers, first responders, ambulance personnel, nurses for the emergency department, critical care physicians, and communication staff?

♦ Were first responders trained in methods of dealing with the special problems of providing medical care during a disaster?

♦ Did the intra-hospital and outside-hospital communication systems have sufficient capacity, flexibility, and backup to enable them to function adequately during the disaster? Specifically, were the following components available: (1) resource management (e.g. dispatch, coordination with EMS, and public services); (2) medical supervision; and

(3) hospital-to-mobile unit and hospital-to-hospital and other public services communication?

◆ Was the equipment required to implement a response available and working?

Process (activities carried out during the disaster period)

Process (activities) refers to the manner in which the system performed during the disaster period. Obviously, this component of the evaluation is essential if the evaluation team and stakeholders are to understand what aspects of the response worked well and what did not go as planned and why. We insist that it is just as important to document what activities were carried out effectively in order to document which planned activities did not transpire in an optional fashion.

Also, it is important to understand what barriers were encountered and how these were addressed, successfully or not.

Examples of process questions follow. They are derived from the response components described in Chapter 4 and also from the logic model (Chapter 7).

◆ How soon did detection, extrication, and medical staff arrive at the disaster scene?

◆ Were detection, extrication, and medical staff able to apply their medical knowledge under disaster conditions? What factors prevented optimum performance?

◆ Did detection, extrication, and medical staff have the skills and knowledge required to perform the functions during a disaster?

◆ How effectively was the triage function performed? What factors interfered?

◆ Was there adequate control over the management and deployment of resources during the disaster? Was responsibility for decision-making clear? Were appropriate decisions made concerning the process of getting patients to appropriate triage and treatment?

◆ How were patients transferred from the scene of the disaster to treatment sites? Was appropriate care provided at the scene?

◆ Were the coordination and communications between hospital and outside hospital units effective in-patient transfers into and out of the hospital or other treatment sites?

◆ How well did hospitals respond to the volume of patients? How well did pre-hospital care units make decisions about on-the-scene treatment and transfer?

- What first aid was provided to victims, by whom, and when? Was this appropriate and effective?
- How did volunteers function? Was their participation supportive or did it interfere with the treatment of patients? What controls, if any, were exercised?
- What compromises in standard medical care were made? Were these compromises acceptable and necessary?
- Was the public prepared to act appropriately when the disaster occurred? What should be added to the public education and information effort in order to facilitate the medical response?
- Was a process undertaken to identify the needs of the affected population? How accurate and timely was the process? Was the information used to support the rescue effort?
- Was the safety and security of the population established and maintained?
- Were food, shelter, and water provided? In a timely manner?
- How effective and accurate were initial communications concerning injury and damage?
- How soon after notification did paramedics/doctors appear at the site of disaster?
- Who (persons and organizations) participated in the response?
- To what extent was the pre-hospital system able to function as designed? How many survivors were turned away/rerouted due to damage to hospital beds, ICU beds, supplies, and staff?
- What types of survivors were cared for? What types were the hospital and pre-hospital systems and field stations unable to serve? For what reasons?
- How effectively did hospitals cooperate to distribute patients in order to share the burden of treatment and to refer patients in need to specialty care? Were there preexisting agreements to this effect? Were these part of a formal preparedness planning process?
- How effective was the coordination among response personnel?
- Was field triage performed?
- Was basic life support administered?
- Was advanced life support provided when required?

Outcomes

Outcome assessment looks at the results of the medical and public health response.

Important outcome questions include:

- What was the extent of disaster related morbidity and mortality?
- Were the immediate health needs of the affected population met? Unmet?
- Did death and/or injury occur that could have been prevented?
- Was the safety of the population adequately secured?
- Were the food needs addressed?
- Were sanitation issues handled effectively?
- Was the affected population appropriately sheltered?
- Was support provided to address the mental health needs of victims and survivors in the short term? Long-term?
- How effective was the triage process?
- How effective was each of the following functions performed?
  - command, control, coordination
  - communications
  - identification of needs
  - search and rescue
  - triage
  - field medical care
  - transport
  - hospital care
  - surge capacity

Each of the above factors could also be examined under the category of 'process' assessment to determine if the functions were actually carried out.

Adequacy

When carrying out an assessment of the adequacy of the response, the evaluation team would want to know the extent to which the total needs of the affected population was met. For example:

- What percentage of the total affected population who required medical assistance actually received it?
- What percentage of the total affected population who required food received needed supplies/were served?
- What percentage of the total affected population who required sanitation assistance had their needs met?

- ◆ What percentage of the total need for triage was met?
- ◆ What percentage of the total need for transport of victims was met?
- ◆ What percentage of the total need for hospital care was met?

The stakeholder group should be able to use these suggestions to target questions of adequacy to the questions of greatest importance to each evaluation group over and above the minimum recommendations.

Monetary Costs

The evaluation of costs related to a disaster response could be addressed on several levels. On the most basic level an evaluation team could develop a total cost for the medical and public health response. Other cost questions could address costs related to each of the components of the response effort. A detailed cost analysis would include the sources of funds, an analysis of whether the money and resources were prioritized in the most effective manner to address the most critical needs, which key response functions were underfunded (and why). Could mutual aid agreements have led to a more timely flow of money and supplies?

Of course 'monetary costs' are only one representation of the expense associated with disaster response; however, it is the most directly available indicator.

Summary

We have offered a rather lengthy set of questions for consideration by a disaster evaluation team and stakeholder group. It is useful to organize these questions into categories that conform to those used in a typical logic model, namely structure (inputs), process (activities), and outcomes, while also addressing adequacy and costs. The sample logic model and the suggested minimum data set which are presented in the chapters that follow should provide guidance to the stakeholder group during their discussions about which issues and questions are most salient for their community's evaluation of the medical and public health response.

References

Ricci, E. and Pretto, E. (1991). Assessment of Prehospital Response in Disasters. *Critical Care Clinics*. 7 (2), pp. 471–493.

Suchman, E. (1967). *Evaluative Research*. New York, NY: Russell Sage Foundation, pp. 60–66.

Further reading

Shaw, I.F., Greene, J.C., and Mark, M.M., eds. (2006). *The Sage Handbook of Evaluation*. Thousand Oaks, CA: Sage.

Wholey, J.S., Hatry, H., and Newcomer, K., eds. (2010) *Handbook of Practical Program Evaluation*, 3rd ed. San Francisco, CA: Josey-Bass (see especially Chapter 1: Planning and Designing Useful Evaluations, pp. 5–29).

Chapter 7

Construct the Logic Model and Research Design (Step 3)

Keypoints

A 'mixed-methods' research design, based upon the categories contained in a disaster response logic model, is suggested as the best approach to capture the complexities of the medical and public health disaster response experience. A mixed-methods design allows the evaluation team to collect and combine data from direct observation, medical records, interviews with victims, health professionals, family and friends of victims, public safety officials, other government and non-governmental officials, and from public documents. Validation in a mixed-method design is based upon the concept of triangulation. The term triangulation is used in behavioral research to describe the process of obtaining data from three or more different sources and then comparing the findings to assess consistency across sources. In this design, both qualitative and quantitative data are collected and then merged during the analysis phase. Each data set is used to validate and enhance the other in order to improve the validity of the conclusions reached and the recommendations that follow. However, not all data need be combined. The mixed-method design allows for the analysis of certain types of data separately and then applied to the appropriate research question because there may be no appropriate comparative data.

Introduction

A detailed research design is an essential component of every scientific evaluation study. The research design should be grounded in a scientific framework and methods that guides the data collection and analysis process. Indeed, evaluators have several such models from which to choose, from highly structured quantitative to less structured observational approaches, and we can find much discussion among evaluation scientists about the strengths and weakness of each. Fortunately, we need not engage in the longstanding debate between 'experimentalists' and those who use other methods because randomized controlled experiments are not possible in disaster evaluations except for certain types of 'preparedness' and engineering studies.

Historically, evaluations conducted of the response to disasters have employed any number of scientific models. We can find in the scientific literature disaster evaluation studies that have used:

- Partial 'case control' or other type of quasi-experimental design, often drawing on medical records to assess disaster related morbidity and mortality.

- Systematic surveys, using a combination of structured and open-ended questions, of responders and members of the affected population.

- In-depth interviews with participants and knowledgeable key informants.

- On-site observations by observers experienced in disaster response combined with analysis of public documents, medical records, and interviews.

- And, of course, any of these methods of data collection can be used in combination with one or more of the others. These are now commonly called mixed-method designs.

Historically, disaster evaluation studies have been carried out by physicians and other clinical specialists, emergency response personnel, epidemiologists, social/behavioral scientists, and, rarely by public health-trained evaluation scientists. As noted in Part 1, scientific disaster evaluation does *not* fall exclusively within the domain of any profession or discipline; rather, it is essentially a complex multidisciplinary endeavor. However, in the future, evaluation scientists should be drawn routinely into disaster evaluation studies because they have familiarity and experience applying the mixed-methods design based upon a logic model described in this field manual.

Logic Model to Guide the Disaster Evaluation Study

As noted in Chapter 3, a logic model describes the resources (inputs), process (activities), outputs, and short-term, intermediate, and long-term outcomes expected to result from an intervention such as a disaster response. As described elsewhere in the book, a logic model may be thought of as a series of 'if–then' statements which, taken as a whole, constitute a program theory that explains how the intervention (disaster response in our situation) is expected to work.

In Figure 7.1, we suggest a basic general logic model for the medical and public health disaster response. This basic logic model contains the essential

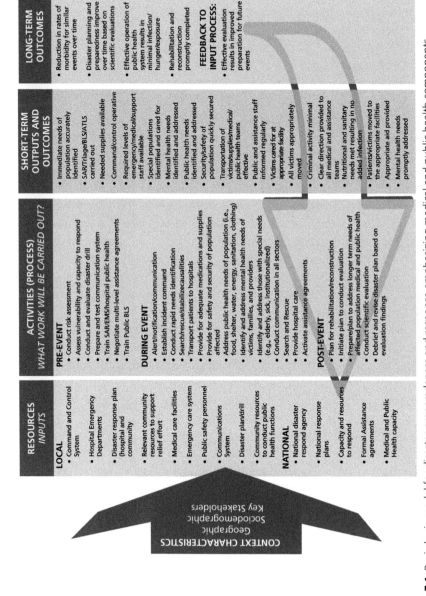

CONTEXT CHARACTERISTICS Geographic Sociodemographic Key Stakeholders	RESOURCES INPUTS	ACTIVITIES (PROCESS) WHAT WORK WILL BE CARRIED OUT?	SHORT-TERM OUTPUTS AND OUTCOMES	LONG-TERM OUTCOMES
	LOCAL • Command and Control System • Hospital Emergency Departments • Disaster response plan (hospital and community) • Relevant community resources to support relief effort • Medical care facilities • Emergency care system • Public safety personnel • Communications System • Disaster plan/drill • Community resources to conduct public health functions **NATIONAL** • National disaster respond agency • National response plans • Capacity and resources to respond • Formal Assistance agreements • Medical and Public Health capacity	**PRE-EVENT** • Conduct risk assessment • Assess vulnerability and capacity to respond • Conduct and evaluate disaster drill • Prepare and test communication system • Train SAR/EMS/hospital public health • Negotiate multi-level assistance agreements • Train Public BLS **DURING EVENT** • Alert/notification/communication • Establish incident command • Conduct rapid needs identification • Search/rescue/stabilize casualties • Transport patients to hospitals • Provide for adequate medications and supplies • Provide for safety and security of population affected • Address public health needs of population (i.e., food, shelter, water, energy, sanitation, clothing) • Identify and address mental health needs of victims, families, and providers • Identify and address those with special needs (e.g., elderly, sick, institutionalized) • Conduct communication in all sectors • Search and Rescue • Provide hospital care • Activate assistance agreements **POST-EVENT** • Plan for rehabilitation/reconstruction • Initiate plan to conduct evaluation • Prepare/plan to address longer term needs of affected population medical and public health • Conduct scientific evaluation • Debrief and revise disaster plan based on evaluation findings	• Immediate needs of population accurately identified • SAR/Triage/BLS/ATLS carried out • Needed supplies available • Command/control operative • Required levels of emergency/medical/support staff available • Special populations identified and cared for • Mental health needs identified and addressed • Public health needs identified and addressed • Security/safety of population quickly secured • Transportation of victims/supplies/medical/ public health teams effective • Public and assistance staff informed regularly • Victims cared for at appropriate facility • All victims appropriately moved • Criminal activity minimal • Clear direction provided to all medical and assistance teams • Nutritional and sanitary needs met resulting in no added infection • Patients/victims moved to the appropriate facilities • Appropriate aid provided • Mental health needs promptly addressed	• Reduction in rates of morbidity for similar events over time • Disaster planning and preparedness improve over time based on scientific evaluations • Effective operation of public health system results in minimal infection/ hunger/exposure • Rehabilitation and reconstruction promptly completed **FEEDBACK TO INPUT PROCESS:** • Effective evaluation results in improved preparation for future events

Figure 7.1 Basic logic model for disaster preparedness and response emphasizing medical and public health components.

elements of a disaster response system. It will serve as the basis for our recommendation (in Chapter 8) of a minimum set of variables that should be considered for inclusion in all medical and public health disaster evaluations and it is offered as a starting point for any future evaluation. We recommend that our suggested logic model be considered a starting point to be modified and adapted to fit the specific circumstances of each disaster and the community(s) in which it occurred.

The logic model presented in Figure 7.1 contains a hypothesized set of essential elements for a medical and public health response to a disaster. In the first column, Resources (also called Inputs), we identify the basic components required for an effective response; the contextual factors are basic indicators of the human and social capital within the affected population. The Activities column is a list of essential activities (the process) that must be carried out promptly during the period in which the event has occurred. These activities are drawn from the description of a response system such as the one described in Chapter 4 of this field manual. The Outputs column identifies the products produced by the activities. The Outcomes columns specify the expected short-term and long-term results to be achieved by the intervention, in this case the medical and public health response.

In Figure 7.1 we have combined into one column short-term outputs with outcomes due to the unique and rapidly changing context within which the disaster response unfolds. In such a situation, some outputs and outcomes may be one and the same.

Once the immediate impacts of the disaster have been addressed, and stabilization has begun within the disaster impact zone, we enter the post-event phase of recovery and rehabilitation. It is then that evaluation is typically begun in earnest. Obviously, the logic model presented here must be adapted to fit the unique situation which is created by each individual disaster and the community context within which the disaster unfolded.

Using the sample logic model shown in Figure 7.1 as a starting point, the evaluation team leader and stakeholder group should adjust it to fit the disaster they are to evaluate. The team should then prepare a detailed set of evaluation questions that should address, at a minimum, the fundamental activities and outcomes that are displayed in the logic model which has been specifically prepared for the evaluation to be undertaken.

Mixed-method Design for Disaster Evaluation

Mixed-methods models have only recently been formalized and described by scientific methodologists and epistemologists. A mixed-method study is characterized by a focus on research problems that require:

- An examination of real life contextual description, multi-level perspectives (individual, organizational, and political jurisdiction), and cultural influences.

- An intentional use of both quantitative data assessing the magnitude and frequency of key factors and qualitative research and information to explore in depth the meaning and understanding of the information gathered during the evaluation.

- A desire to draw upon the strengths of quantitative and qualitative data in order to formulate a holistic interpretive framework generating possible solutions or new understandings of the intervention being evaluated. (adapted from Creswell et al., 2003).

Drawing upon the comments of several methodologists, a team at the University of Southern California identified several advantages associated with the use of mixed-method designs. Among the strengths of these designs are:

- Narrative and non-textual information can add meaning to numeric data, while numeric data can add precision to narrative ... information.

- Can utilize existing data while at the same time generating and testing a program theory.

- A broader, more complex research problem can be investigated because the researcher is not constrained by using only one method.

- The strengths of one method can be used to overcome the inherent weaknesses of the other method.

- Can provide stronger more robust evidence to support a conclusion or set of recommendations.

- May generate new knowledge, new insights or uncover hidden insights, patterns, or relationships that a single methodological approach might not reveal.

- Produces more complete knowledge and understanding of the research problem that can be used to ... (advance) theory or practice.

(adapted from Tashakkori and Teddlie, 2003)

However, mixed-methods designs can present complex problems during the analysis stage when qualitative data are either merged or examined separately and then compared with numeric data. We will offer an approach to handling these problems in Chapter 12. Also, implementing a mixed-method design virtually mandates that a multidisciplinary evaluation team be assembled because few individuals are sufficiently trained in both quantitative and qualitative methods and designs to manage the inherent complexities of collecting and analyzing both types of data.

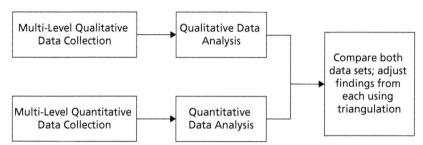

Figure 7.2 Triangulation design: multi-level congruence design for merged data sets.

The mixed-method design we propose for disaster evaluation studies is called a 'triangulation: multi-level congruent design' (Tashakkori and Teddlie, 2003). The model is shown in Figure 7.2. Although the label is imposing, the meaning of the design is quite straightforward and intuitive. Basically, this design instructs the research team to collect both qualitative and quantitative data as separate processes and then compare and merge the data where appropriate or, present each type of data separately when that is sufficient to answer the evaluative question being addressed.

In using this design, researchers collect both quantitative and qualitative data about individuals, organizations, and systems that were affected by the disaster and use each data set to validate and enhance understandings obtained from the other. This design leads to a more valid, and better substantiated set of findings, conclusions, and recommendations than would be possible with any other type of design.

Non-merged Data

However, it is important to note that not all data in a mixed-method design should or can be merged. Much of the data stands alone as, for example, quantitative counts of such factors as number who died or were injured (often reported by location and cause) or qualitative (textual quotes) reports of personal experiences of victims. Obviously, it is appropriate to report these categories of information without merging and comparing them.

Our proposed mixed-method design requires (1) obtaining data from multiple sources, namely medical records, structured interviews with public officials, victims/family members, bystanders, first responders and participating non-governmental organization staff, and from relevant documents; (2) pre-prepared data collection instruments which contain the minimum data set as defined in this field manual; (3) a scientific sampling plan; (4) a

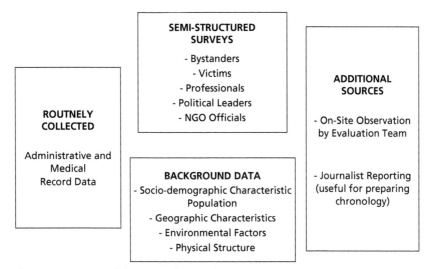

Figure 7.3 Sources of disaster evaluation data.

multi-disciplinary evaluation team; and (5) an appropriate stakeholder group that works with an evaluation study project director.

In Figure 7.3 we summarize the many sources from which data, both quantitative and qualitative, are likely to be obtained in a comprehensive disaster evaluation study.

Summary

In this chapter we have provided a detailed example of a logic model that can be used and adapted as necessary by future evaluation teams and stakeholder groups to create a 'theory' of how the response effort should have functioned, i.e. the resources and context for the evaluation, the activities to be carried out, and the expected outputs and outcomes. Each of the variables contained in the logic model should be measured/assessed after the sample logic model has been adjusted to the specifics of each individual disaster to which it will be applied. The research design will require a mixed-methods approach which allows for the collection of both process and outcome data in qualitative and quantitative formats.

Reference

Creswell, J., Plano Clark, V.L., Guttinann, M.T., and Hanson, W. (2003). Advanced mixed methods designs. In: Tashakkori, A. and Teddlie, C., eds., *Handbook of Mixed Methods in Social and Behavioral Research*, 1st ed. Thousand Oaks, CA: Sage Publications, pp. 209–240.

Further reading

Creswell, J.W. and **Clark, V.P.** (2018). *Designing and Conducting Mixed Methods Research*, 3rd ed. Thousand Oaks, CA: Sage Publications.

Donaldson, S.I., Christie, C.A., and **Mark, M.,** eds. (2015). *Credible and Actionable Evidence*, 2nd ed. Thousand Oaks, CA: Sage Publications, p. VII.

Datta, L. (1997). Multi-method evaluations: Using case studies together with other methods. In: **Chelimsky, E.** and **Shadish, W.,** eds., *Evaluation for the 21st Century, A Handbook*. Thousand Oaks, CA: Sage Publications, pp. 349–359.

Chapter 8

Prepare Mixed-method Data Collection Instruments (Step 4)

Keypoints

This chapter builds upon the response system components described in Chapter 4 and the logic model presented in Chapter 7. The stakeholder group that is assembled to guide the evaluation should determine the evaluation questions that are of greatest interest to them. Topical interview guides are typically prepared to guide interviews with professional responders, victims (or their surrogates), public health, safety, and governmental administrators, and non-governmental organization participants. In addition, an autopsy/hospital record abstract form and an 'observation guide' are often included in the set of data collection forms. Data collection forms used in past evaluations can be found in Appendix C and may be useful as examples.

Minimum (Basic) Set of Variables (Data) For Medical and Public Health Response Evaluations

Drawing upon the components of a disaster response system described in Chapter 4 and our sample logic model, we have identified a minimum (basic) set of variables and data elements that should be considered for inclusion in disaster evaluation studies whose goal is to assess how the medical and public health system performed, and the outcomes achieved, throughout the disaster impact period. These indicators are presented in Table 8.1. We recommend that data concerning each of these variables be considered by the stakeholder group and the evaluation team for inclusion in the evaluation study. The 'Before Disaster Event' variables will provide context within which the response activities occurred and outcomes reached (or not). The 'During Event' variables are displayed into those that reflect the emergency system operation and victim

Table 8.1 Minimum (basic) set of variables for inclusion in disaster evaluation studies

Before disaster event	During disaster event	After disaster event
Socio-economic characteristics of disaster region ◆ Per capita income ◆ Median income: individual/family ◆ Under 5 infant mortality rates ◆ Life expectancy: male, female ◆ GDP per capita ◆ % population homeless ◆ Median adult education: male, female ◆ % population access to potable water ◆ % population rural/urban ◆ Population density/size/by age **Health/public health system** ◆ Physicians per capita ◆ Hospital beds per capita ◆ Level of EMS system development ◆ Health care workers per capita ◆ Number/location of hospitals **Disaster preparedness** ◆ Completed assessment of hazards and their risk factors ◆ Disaster plan completed ◆ Disaster drill completed	**Emergency system operation level** ◆ Type of event; magnitude; scale; size of affected population; geographic area affected ◆ Needs identification study conducted: Yes/No? Accurate? Time completed? ◆ Capability of health organizations within impact area to respond ◆ Communication with public: How? Reach? Clarity? ◆ Operation of incident command system ◆ Availability of medical supplies/supply chain management ◆ Barriers encountered during the emergency response? Were these barriers addressed? How were they addressed? ◆ Time to first response team arrival ◆ Time to declaration of disaster ◆ Effectiveness of triage/ search and rescue **Victim Level (from sample of victims)** ◆ Name ◆ Age and gender ◆ Type and severity of injury or illness ◆ Date and time of injury and rescue ◆ Location of victim when injured ◆ Location of provided treatment provided. At scene? During transport? At hospital? ◆ Final diagnosis of injury ◆ Role of bystanders and family ◆ Effectiveness of triage ◆ How transported to treatment ◆ Final patient outcome	**Public health system level** ◆ Sanitation needs met? ◆ Housing, food, clothing, potable water provided? ◆ Activity of relief organizations: name, type, contribution ◆ Describe overall coordination of relief effort ◆ Availability of needed medical supplies, equipment, and resources ◆ Major barriers encountered during post event period: Resolved or unresolved? ◆ Disaster-related infections/disease/ surveillance/control ◆ Mental health issues identified and addressed? ◆ Needs of special populations (e.g. elderly, physically handicapped, mentally handicapped) addressed? ◆ Operation of medical treatment facilities **Region/community level** ◆ Infrastructure damage that could affect public health ◆ Operation of medical treatment facilities ◆ Ongoing communication with public ◆ Final count of disaster-related deaths and injuries ◆ Number of affected persons in disaster zone ◆ Electric power generation ◆ Mass fatality management

level data. The 'After disaster' public health system and the regional/community level variables are designed to reveal the full impact of the disaster, and to some extent the resilience of the population affected, within the geographic region struck by the disaster.

Sample Data Collection Forms

The sample data collection forms shown in Appendix C are provided with several goals in mind. They have been used in past studies of earthquake-related injury and mortality; however, they only serve as a starting point for future disaster evaluation studies.

First, at this time in the evolution of disaster evaluation studies, it will be useful to compare and contrast the preparation, response, and outcomes identified with similar types of disasters in order to identify the correlates and, hopefully, the causes of successful or inadequate response.

Secondly, the preparation of data collection forms that will provide valid and reliable data is a formidable technical task. It can be very time consuming. The forms we offer have been used in several disaster studies, and each use has led to modification and improvement of the forms.

Thirdly, it is obviously important to begin the data collection process as quickly as possible; having data collection forms 'ready to go' will greatly shorten the time to the beginning of data collection. This is especially critical if concurrent data collection is possible and attempted. In situations where concurrent data collection is initiated it would not be possible to proceed without the availability of pre-prepared data collection forms.

Finally, if we stay true to the logic contained in our logic model both process and outcome data must be collected if we are to develop a comprehensive understanding of the response effort. Having data collection forms in hand will guide the research team to collect both categories of data. The forms are offered only as guidance for an evaluation team. They may be used in full or modified to fit the unique circumstances of each disaster because they were originally designed for use in assessing the response to earthquakes.

Suggestions for the Construction of Data Collection Forms

Data collection for disaster evaluation studies is carried out using four primary methods; (1) guided observations using checklists and observation guides; (2) group or individual interviews with victims or their surrogates using structured questionnaires for individuals or discussion guides for group interviews;

(3) interviews with professional health and public health workers and others (governmental or non-governmental organization officials, public safety personnel); and (4) abstract forms to guide data collection from existing health records and from public data sources. These primary methods may be supplemented with group interviews using a 'focus group' process, public records including newspaper accounts (good source of dates as to when events occurred), and agency reports of meetings held to discuss the disaster response.

Questionnaires

Two types of questionnaires are used in disaster evaluation studies. *Structured (fixed response)* questionnaires provide the respondent with a set of response options for each question. Structured questionnaires have several advantages. First, the evaluation team can be certain that the respondent is considering the full range of possible answers before providing an answer. Secondly, the responses are more easily and quickly converted to quantitative data than is possible with more open-ended questions. Thirdly, following the conversion to quantitative data more complex statistical analysis is possible.

Semi-structured or open-ended questions allow the respondent more flexibility to respond and to more fully express feeling, attitudes or descriptions of events, barriers, unusual events or processes, etc. These less structured questions are valuable when the evaluation team wants to expand and deepen the understanding of what occurred during the disaster response. Often a mixture of both fixed response and semi-structured or open-ended questions are employed.

Focus Group

The focus group process involves the simultaneous interview of up to six to eight persons who are carefully selected for the perspective they can provide. The focus group leader uses a set of pre-determined questions or topics to guide the discussion. This process encourages the expression of varying viewpoints, opinions, and beliefs about each topic and, guided properly, can lead to a fuller description of the disaster response effort. The participants can stimulate one another thus aiding recall, debate different points of view until consensus is reached, and draw out individuals who may be reluctant to speak in a one-to-one setting. Typically the members of a focus group are homogeneous along one or more personal characteristics (e.g. all public safety personnel or, all victims and family members of the victims). The homogeneity tends to increase the comfort level of the participants and it brings a common vocabulary and background to the discussion. (Hennick, 2013).

Focus groups, if conducted in an environment in which the participants feel comfortable, are a highly cost-effective method of collecting information about the disaster experience. Typically, the goal in a focus group interview, is not to obtain consensus about a topic or issue, although that may naturally occur. It is, rather, to obtain a full range of opinion or, the broad experience of the participants, relative to a particular topic or event.

One interesting characteristic of focus groups is worth mentioning. In a focus group, participants are free to interact with each other. This has the unique effect of refining the statements of opinion and observation of each member of the group which serves as a form of quality check on the information provided. Such a benefit is only available through a collective response process such as provided by a focus group.

Chronology of Disaster-related Events

We strongly recommend that a detailed chronology of events, showing day and approximate time and sequence for each, be constructed to describe the most important disaster-related events from the start of the event and through the four-week period after the start. A detailed chronology can be of great value in visualizing how the disaster unfolded, how the response teams attempted to meet the challenges as they unfolded, what barriers they encountered, and how these were dealt with. Data for the chronology can be obtained from interviews with key decision-makers who directed the response, from newspaper accounts and from other public records.

While newspaper accounts may or may not be thoroughly validated, they are typically quite accurate as to when events did occur. They are usually accessible from the newspaper archives or on-line. The chronology will be of great value when the evaluation team prepares findings and recommendations because it will highlight events and activities to focus upon where the response worked well and where barriers were encountered.

Why Collect Data for All Categories of the Logic Model?

We suggest that evaluation studies be based upon data collected for all categories of the logic model. Without an understanding of how the response system performed (activities/process) and the resources available (inputs/structure) it is difficult if not impossible to explain how it came about that the desired outcomes were or were not achieved. Or, put in program evaluation terms, it will not be possible to use the program theory as described in the logic model to acquire a comprehensive understanding of the disaster preparedness and response effort.

A Comment About Concurrent Data Collection and Evaluation

We are aware of attempts to establish and test a system by which certain data could be collected by one or more members of an evaluation team during the disaster event. In concurrent data collection the data collection team would pre-arrange to enter the disaster zone with first-responder teams, collect observations using structured checklists and free-formed impressions, and conduct structured interviews with first responders, family members of victims, and victims where possible as the response effort is unfolding.

In addition, much data and relevant information is now created as disasters unfold. This includes (1) record keeping by medical personnel; (2) video recordings of the event by on the scene broadcast journalists; (3) journalistic reporting on-site; and (4) cell phone communication and picture taking by those who are within the disaster impact area and are thereby experiencing the disaster as it unfolds. Methods for the inclusion of concurrent data collection are likely to evolve and be routinely employed in future evaluation studies.

Summary

When preparing data for a disaster preparedness and response evaluation, team members may draw upon the data collection forms provided in Appendix C and the basic set of variables identified in Table 8.1. The basic variables and the sample forms provided in this book should be modified to fit the unique circumstances of each individual disaster. However, we suggest that the logic model and data set prepared for each disaster evaluation include the basic components of a disaster response system and that the data collection forms contain questions directed at measuring each of the essential variables contained in the logic model which was used to plan the evaluation study.

Reference

Hennick, M. (2013). *Focus Group Discussions*. London: Oxford University Press, p. 3.

Further reading

Bourque, L.B., Siegel, J.M., and Kano, M.M. (2007). Morbidity and mortality associated with disasters. In: *Handbook of Disaster Research*. Rodriguez, H., Quaraentelli, E.L., and Dynes, R.R., eds. New York, NY: Springer, pp. 97–112.

Checchi, F. and Roberts, L. (2008). Documenting Mortality in Crisis: What Keeps us From Doing Better? *PLOS Medicine*. 5 (7), e146.

Debacker, M., Hubloue, I., Dhondt, E., et al. (2012). Utstein-Style Template For Uniform Data Reporting of Acute Medical Response in Disasters. *PLOS Currents.* 4, e4f6cf3e8df15a.

Stratton S.J. (2012). The Utstein-Style Template for Uniform Data Reporting of Acute Medical Response in Disasters. *Prehospital and Disaster Medicine.* 27 (**3**), p. 219.

U.S. Centers For Disease Control and Prevention. (2018). *Public Health Surveillance During a Disaster.* Atlanta, GA: U.S. Centers For Disease Control and Prevention.

Chapter 9

Construct a Sampling Plan (Step 5)

Keypoints

In disaster studies it is necessary to obtain information from several groups of those involved and affected by the disaster and from various types of medical and administrative documents. We have suggested in Chapter 8 that information be obtained from, at a minimum, (1) survivors/victims/families; (2) professional responders and coordinators (both public safety and EMS/medical); (3) officials of governmental and non-governmental organizations; (4) medical records; and (5) administrative documents. This typically involves accessing a large number of individuals and reports. It is therefore almost always necessary to select a sample from each group and source. When possible some form of random (probability) sampling should be used; a different type of sampling called 'purposive' may be employed for key informants. 'Convenience samples' are not generally used in scientific evaluation studies due to their great potential for introducing bias into the data. Preparing and implementing a scientific sample design will prove to be one of the most challenging aspects of disaster evaluation studies. It will usually be necessary to consult with an individual who has statistical expertise when preparing the sampling plan; therefore, in this chapter we present some basic concepts in sampling and then conclude with four descriptions of sample designs used in past evaluation studies.

Introduction to Sampling for Disaster Evaluations: Definitions of Basic Terms

Owing to cost and time constraints it is seldom possible, nor is it necessary, to obtain data from all participants, and from the totality of administrative and medical records, for any mass-casualty disaster; therefore, scientific sampling techniques must be employed by the evaluation team. Scientific sampling methods allow evaluators to draw conclusions about the totality of the disaster event, and the medical and public health response, with a high degree of certainty that their findings and conclusions are correct. A sample is a subgroup (subset) of a population whose characteristics are studied to gain information about the whole population.

It follows that selecting a sample is the process of identifying a group to represent the members of the total population from which it is drawn. If selected using scientific statistical methodology, the sample will closely mirror the characteristics of the population from which it is drawn. Obtaining a census, which is an enumeration of the total population of interest, is obviously, more costly, time consuming, and more difficult if not impossible in disaster conditions. It is also unnecessary given the accuracy that can be achieved by applying scientific sampling methods.

Approaches to Sampling for Disaster Studies

There are two general approaches to scientific sampling for evaluation studies, namely 'random' and 'non-random', both of these must be used in comprehensive evaluation studies. In *random sampling* every information unit (individual or record) from the total number of units in the area affected by the disaster will be equally likely to be included. For example, if the evaluation team wants to assess the medical help provided to all those who were injured (i.e. the *total population* of victims), it would not be necessary to interview and examine the medical record of every one of those injured; or, if one wanted to obtain the views of all emergency responders or physicians who participated in the search, rescue, and initial treatment effort, a sample would be sufficient.

The second approach is called *purposive sampling*. In purposive sampling, we identify key informants who, due to their formal position (political leader, head of NGO, director of local hospital, etc.), have a unique perspective and therefore should be interviewed. We discuss each type of sample in the sections that follow.

Random Samples

There are several types of random sample designs available to an evaluation team.

Systematic Random Sample

To prepare a 'systematic random sample' it is necessary to have a randomly ordered list of the units (persons, records, etc.) to be examined. The list is called a *sampling frame.* Then, using a predetermined pattern of selection, every person or record in the unit is selected for inclusion in the study. For example, every fifth person or record would be identified for inclusion in the study. A variation to a systematic random sample is a process in which the units to be sampled are selected using a random technique such as drawing names from a box of names, or using a table of random members.

Stratified Random Sampling

This refers to the process of sorting the units to be sampled into groups called strata and then randomly sampling from each group. Stratification is useful when the groups from which data are to be obtained vary in size, and the evaluation team wants to make certain that information is obtained from each subgroup.

Cluster Random Sampling

Cluster random sampling refers to the procedure of identifying naturally occurring clusters of the units to be examined. Such clusters may be blocks in a city, communities, schools, hospitals, census tracts, for example. In cluster random sampling, the first step (stage) is to randomly select a sample of 'clusters' and then, either proportionately or non-proportionately, select a sample of units to be included in the study. Cluster random sampling has the great advantage of allowing data collection to occur more efficiently and at less cost than is possible with the other sample designs because the units to be included in the study (for example individuals or records) are located in close proximity.

Multi-stage Sample

Multi-stage sampling involves selecting a sample in two or more stages. For example, in the *first* stage large units (often geographic, e.g. counties, provinces) or clusters of the population who share a quality of interest such as their distance or proximity to a disaster impact zone. In the *second* stage one might select blocks of houses within each first stage cluster. A *third* stage, if needed, could involve the selection of individual houses within the blocks. Multi-stage samples are widely used in public health research of all types. They are useful when it is costly or virtually impossible to prepare a list of all units to be sampled in the target area. Although a multi-stage sample typically gives less precise estimates than a simple random sample of the same size it is a far more cost-effective approach to obtain statistically valid data and the estimates obtained are usually more than adequate to answer disaster evaluation questions.

Non-random Samples

Purposive samples are not selected on the basis of each unit (person, house, block, etc.) having an 'equal probability of inclusion'. Rather, the evaluation team selects these participants or records for the unique perspective they may provide due to the nature of their participation in the response or because they experienced something rare, unusual, or limited in some way. For example the evaluation team might want to examine closely those victims who were severely injured, but were among the last rescued; or look in depth into the experience of the hospitals that cared for the first wave of victims. Usually, an evaluation team will interview each individual who played a key role in implementing the response. Also, key political leaders may be included in the study if they were involved in the preparedness and/or response.

Purposive samples are identified because they are expected to lead to an in depth understanding of one or more of the research questions, whereas random sampling techniques are used when it is desired to specify with precision the experience of the total population of those affected by the population.

The difference is explained by Kemper et al.:

'The logic and power of purposive sampling lies in selecting information-rich cases for study in depth' (Patton, 1990, p. 169), with an underlying focus on intentionally selecting specific cases that will provide the most information for the questions under study. Researchers using random sampling techniques often seek to maximize the sample size so as to increase the probability of making accurate generalizations from the data. In contrast, researchers using purposive techniques seek to focus and, where practical, minimize the sample size, generally in nonrandom ways, so as to select only those cases that might best illuminate and test the hypothesis of the research team. Although purposive sampling techniques are commonly associated with qualitative methods, purposive sampling can be used within studies with either a qualitative or quantitative orientation and are quite common in mixed methods studies.

(Kemper et al., 2003)

Quota Samples

Quota samples, another form of non-random sample, are also useful in disaster evaluation studies. In quota sampling interviewers select respondents until a pre-determined number of individuals in pre-determined categories is reached. One might, for example, decide that given limited availability of funds to conduct the evaluation, it is only possible to interview 100 individuals in the disaster zone. A decision may be made to spread the interviewer as follows: 30 victim survivors; 30 family members of victims who died; 15 search and rescue personnel; ten physicians; 15 emergency care responders.

In both purposive and quota samples the research team cannot quantitatively calculate the 'precision' of the information provided. Here, precision is used in the statistical sense to mean closeness of estimates under repeated estimates of the same size. Judgment is therefore required to assess the extent to which these samples can be relied upon to reflect the opinion of the total population of each group about the reality of the disaster response.

Guidelines for Preparing a Sample Design for Disaster Response Evaluations

Sampling Affected Populations

We recommend that data for disaster evaluations that focus on the medical and public health response be obtained from (1) structured interviews with victims or their surrogates; (2) responders both professional and lay to include search and rescue and emergency medical personnel; (3) police and military; (4) public officials who directed and coordinated the response; (5) citizens who reside in the disaster area (random sample); (6) staff of NGOs that participated (purposive sample); (7) physicians and administrative personnel in hospitals that cared for the victims (purposive sample); (8) medical records such as autopsy reports, individual medical case reports for survivors, and hospital data that reveal the impact of the disaster event (random sample); and (9) data about structural damage to buildings (purposive sample).

This information is most appropriately gathered from samples of those individuals affected by the event, from medical records, and from those who participated in the response. The interview and medical record data can be combined with background information about the population, geographic area, preparedness, building vulnerability, etc., which will be obtained from existing sources.

We propose that a grid be overlaid on a map of the disaster area. The grid may be divided into three equal zones (geographic strata) starting with the area of initial or greatest impact and extending to the outer perimeter of impact. Then samples may be drawn of each respondent group within in each zone (refer to Figure 9.1).

In Figure 9.1 we illustrate two disaster sampling situations. In Plan A, we represent the situation in which the disaster damage radiates out from a point of impact. In this case the sample zones are in concentric circles around and extending outward from the point of impact as in an earthquake, explosion, or volcanic eruption.

In Plan B, the sampling zones are equal in size throughout the disaster area, e.g. an island or large city devastated by an intense hurricane or fire.

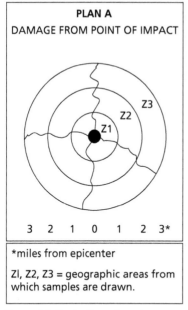
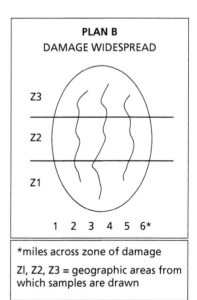

PLAN A

DAMAGE FROM POINT OF IMPACT

3 2 1 0 1 2 3*

*miles from epicenter

Zl, Z2, Z3 = geographic areas from which samples are drawn.

PLAN B

DAMAGE WIDESPREAD

1 2 3 4 5 6*

*miles across zone of damage

Zl, Z2, Z3 = geographic areas from which samples are drawn

Figure 9.1 Illustration of random sampling schematics.

Determination of Sample Size for the Survey (Random) Component

Determining the sample size for an assessment of victim characteristics and outcomes of victims and medical records involves several considerations. The *first* consideration is what is technically called 'confidence level'. Confidence level refers to a rather simple idea as expressed by the question: How much confidence do we have that the individuals interviewed (or represented by medical records) actually represent all the victims?

Several factors can affect the level of confidence. The size of the sample selected is an important determinant of the degree of confidence we have that it is truly representative of the population from which it is selected. Another factor in assessing confidence is the extent to which the sample has been *randomly selected*. Typically, researchers desire confidence levels of 90% or 95% meaning that if we drew 100 random samples of sufficient size we would get the same results 90% of the time or 95% of the time. A third factor is the actual level of response, i.e. the 'response rate'. A low response (often less than 70–80%) could lead to important biases reflected in the data.

In summary, *sampling error*, defined as the difference between the characteristics of the sample and the population from which it was selected, can occur from chance (we just by chance select cases not representative of the total) or from sampling bias. A biased sample can result from a low response or, by favoring some members of the population over others (e.g. those most easy to reach or communicate with).

When the evaluation team and stakeholder group begin a discussion of sampling we strongly suggest that a statistician, or a social scientist who has a background in sampling theory, be consulted. However, some general guidance follows.

- We are always balancing the amount of statistical error we can tolerate with the costs associated with reducing that error, thereby increasing confidence in the findings.

- For populations of up to 20,000, randomly drawn samples of approximately 350 will provide confidence up to the level of 95%. In fact, this confidence level does not change for even significantly higher populations. However, funding to obtain samples of this size is often difficult in disaster evaluation.

- If lower levels of confidence can be tolerated, the sample size may be dramatically reduced. For example, a sample of 200 individuals will produce statistical confidence levels of approximately 80%. However, it is important to note that much of value can be learned from even smaller samples.

- Sample size calculators are readily available online.

Informant Selection for the Purposive Sample

The identification and mapping of informants to be interviewed is a systematic process. The mapping process begins when the liaison person is contacted (usually by the scout team) and proceeds through a series of steps that are described.

- The initial list of persons to be interviewed is derived from the liaison person who identifies the key persons involved in the disaster preparedness and response activity in his/her community/region, and the country, usually during the scout team visit.

- This list is expanded and developed according to a set of categories that contain the key roles/positions that are relevant to the response. These categories may include the EMS regional coordinator, local politicians (city, rural, state, county), person(s) responsible for disaster preparedness, emergency department physicians and nurses (in key hospitals), hospital administrators/planners, ambulance providers, media persons, health department representatives (state and local), public safety officials (police, fire), community representatives (especially minority), regional planning groups (health or other), emergency service personnel (paramedics, nurses), other involved individuals/organizations (military, NGOs).

This list can be developed by using materials from newspaper or other documentary data, and from key informants.

Choices are then made from these lists of interview candidates since the constraints of the field research time may not allow for more than 15–20 interviews to be scheduled initially, and it is necessary to allow the researchers some flexibility to permit the scheduling of additional appointments while in the field. The selection process is based on an issue-specific reputational technique in which the most visible informants in the community identify others until there is significant repetition of the names mentioned, thereby forming the basic list of persons to be interviewed. During the field visit, recommendations from persons interviewed may expand this list and require that additional interviews be scheduled.

The selection of the informants from the master list can also be based on criteria other than the role or position the individuals hold. Temporal, spatial, and social categories are additional selection criteria for interview candidates. For example, older adults may be selected because of their historical knowledge of the social and political community context which may have created barriers to disaster preparedness and/or response. Persons of varying positional status may be chosen so that perspectives from all social and political strata are explored. A range of informants from urban, suburban, and rural contexts or regional extremes, should also be included.

We offer in the next section descriptions of sample designs that have been used in past disaster studies in order to illustrate various approaches to sample design.

Four Examples to Illustrate Approaches to Sample Design

Example 1: Sampling design for study of an earthquake in Turkey

Descriptive epidemiologic, engineering, organizational, displaced persons, and response personnel data were gathered from local government sources and combined with demographic and geographical information to devise and overall sampling plan of the earthquake-affected population. Interviews included lay survivors, search and rescue (SAR) workers (police and military), medical personnel, and local disaster response coordinators. The lay public sample was chosen randomly based on a geographically stratified sampling design. The latter three groups were chosen by tracing each of the major organizations involved in the response effort and interviewing a sample of these personnel.

To facilitate random sampling of lay respondents while ensuring adequate geographic representation of the region, the city and surrounding villages were divided into quadrants (Figure 2). In areas of the city where building damage had been minimal, survivors remained in their homes. In areas of heavier damage, city officials had authorized bulldozing of property and survivors were rehoused in temporary shelters. Each quadrant of the city was divided by street and house or by row and shelter, depending upon the number of remaining, occupied buildings. Dwellings were selected using specific procedures based on total numbers. For example, in each camp, every third shelter was selected for sampling and one household member was interviewed. To reduce any potential bias of obtaining interviews only from the heads of each household, sequential sampling of different household members was used. Thus, at the first home or shelter, the husband was interviewed, at the second, the wife, and at the third, the eldest child if ≥15 years of age. Procedures also were established for incidences when no one was at home in a selected dwelling.

In sampling the rural population, villages with high mortality rates were selected. Therefore, prior to the survey, villages were listed by number of deaths and sorted by quadrants. Within each quadrant, one village was selected at random from among the five with the highest mortality rates ... The head of each village and the relations of residents who had died were interviewed.

Of the 500 police officers who responded to the earthquake, 150 remained in the city. First, the senior police officer involved in the response was interviewed, and then seven others were selected at random. A similar approach was used at the nearby military base for those military personnel who had responded.

Significant destruction to medical facilities in the city had killed many health-care workers. Of those who survived, many left the region and were untraceable. Each remaining hospital in the city was visited, and the most senior physician-administrator as well as physicians and nurses who had been involved in the response also were interviewed. In addition, the senior physician-administrator and chief surgical and medical officers at the main university hospital in the neighboring city of Erzurum were questioned. They had been responsible for the care of the critically ill patients transported out of Erzincan. A sample of government and non-government officials both locally in Erzincan and within the Turkish government in Ankara, also were interviewed.

(Pretto et al., 1994)

Example 2: Sampling design for an assessment of mortality after the 2003 invasion of Iraq

As a first stage of sampling, 50 clusters were selected systematically by governorate with a population proportional to size approach, on the basis of the 2004 UNDP/ Iraqi Ministry of Planning population estimates (table 2). At the second stage of sampling, the Governorate's constituent administrative units were listed by population or estimated population, and location(s) were selected randomly proportionate to population size. The third stage consisted of random selection of a main street within the administrative unit from a list of all main streets. A residential street was then randomly selected from a list of residential streets crossing the main street. On the residential street, houses were outnumbered and a start household was randomly selected. From this start household, the team proceeded to the adjacent residence until 40 households were surveyed. For this study, a household was defined as a unit that ate together and had a separate entrance from the street or a separate apartment entrance.

(Burnham,G., Lafta, R., Doocy, S. and Robert S., 2006)

Example 3: Sampling design for a qualitative study

The method of measurement used in this qualitative study was in-depth interviews using a semi-structured form consisting of three main topics: a) participants' experience in disasters, b) training related to disasters and c) ethical problems encountered during disasters. Interviews were carried out by the first two authors, MMC and KV, in six cities of Turkey; Istanbul, Ankara, Izmir, Bursa, Adana, and Antakya. The first five are the largest cities and have also been exposed to major disasters and have most of the experienced relief workers working in various institutions. Antakya was chosen because it is one of the cities most affected by the migration crisis and war in Syria, and its hospitals have had to face the heavy burden of treating wounded members of armed groups.

A purposeful sampling based on a maximum variation method was chosen in order to reach HCWs (health care workers) with diverse professional backgrounds and experienced in various types of disasters. Another criterion for determining the number of participants was saturation of information. Considering these criteria, 33 HCWs were determined by a snowball sampling technique starting from the disaster response team members of the Turkish Medical Association and Ministry of Health, two of whom declined to participate to the study considering the political dimension of the questions. Therefore 31 HCWs were interviewed between March–May 2014, including physicians whose specialties were general practice, public health, pediatrics, pediatric surgery, cardiovascular surgery, general surgery, psychiatry, anesthesiology and reanimation and medical education. Also, a nurse, a psychologist and two medical students were interviewed.

(Civaner et al., 2017)

Example 4: A cluster survey design employed following a hurricane

Two months after Hurricane Andrew struck Dade County Florida, Health officials conducted a cluster survey to (1) determine the distribution of displaced persons in the county, (2) estimate health needs, (3) gauge access to health and social services, and (4) assess evacuation behaviors. To establish a sampling frame, survey personnel divided Dade County into 6 zones on the basis of damage sustained in each zone. In an attempt to make the sample self-weighting (a statistical technique that simplifies calculation of survey estimates) the officials selected, with probability proportional to size, 30 census tracts in each of the 6 zones. Within each cluster, 10 households were consecutively selected, using a random start. The data were analyzed by using CSAMPLE, a software module of Epi Info (CDC, Atlanta Georgia).

(Wetterhall and Noji, 1997)

A Comment About the 2017 Hurricane in Puerto Rico (Maria)

The September 2017 hurricane that struck the island of Puerto Rico (Maria) presented an opportunity to further refine disaster evaluation methods. Maria was a category 4 hurricane that brought sustained winds of 155 miles per hour—almost reaching the 157 mile per hour level of a category 5. The entire island lost electrical power and communications capability and flooding was experienced throughout. The initial 'official' mortality count was ten later raised to 64. However, to participants in the relief effort and to island residents, that number was not credible.

As a result, the governor of Puerto Rico, seeking an independent estimate of mortality, engaged the George Washington University Milken School of Public Health to conduct a scientific study in order to provide answers to three questions. One of the questions asked for an estimate of hurricane-related mortality. The other study questions directed the research team to assess the quality of the crisis related communication and of the US Centers for Disease Control and prevention guidelines for mortality assessment and reporting in disaster situations. To address the question concerning hurricane-related mortality the study team developed an independent estimate of mortality by conducting a survey of 3,299 randomly selected households during which they asked about displacement, infrastructure loss, and causes of death within the household during the hurricane period. They then compared the estimate obtained from the survey with 'observed mortality' drawn from vital statistics records and with historic mortality rates for the same time period for each year from 2010 to 2017. Using statistical modelling techniques the George Washington team estimated that the true hurricane Maria–related death rate for the post hurricane period was 'using the migration displacement scenario . . . estimated to be 2975 (95% CI:2658– 3290) . . . for the post disaster period' (Milken Institute School of Public Health Final Project Report, 2018).

We call attention to this important study because it contains a creative and useful method of estimating disaster-related mortality which any disaster evaluation team may want to adopt, especially in situations in which the 'official' counts are not in line with observed reality. The method is described in detail in the final project report by the George Washington University Team.

Summary

These sampling plans used in four disaster studies illustrate the basic principles to be followed in preparing a sampling plan. These can be summarized as follows.

- The two basic approaches to sampling, random and non-random, each have utility in every disaster evaluation study.
- A random sample should be used to assess the effects of the disaster, at both time of impact and follow up periods, upon the population affected as revealed in interviews and medical records.

- Purposive sampling may be used to identify key informants who can describe and discuss aspects of the preparedness and rescue activities (the input and activities sections of the logic model).

- Final sample size determination for the random component is dependent upon a number of factors. A statistician or social scientist should be involved in the process.

Acknowledgments

The extract from Pretto et al. 1994 is reproduced with permission from Pretto, Ernesto A. et al., An Analysis of Prehospital Mortality in an Earthquake, Prehospital and Disaster Medicine, 9 (2): pp. 107–117 © World Association for Disaster and Emergency Medicine 1994. doi.org/10.1017/S1049023X00041005. The extract from Kemper E. et al., Mixed Methods Sampling Strategies in Social Research. In: Tashakkori, A. and Teddlie, C., eds., *Handbook of Mixed Methods in Social and Behavioral Research,* pp. 279–280. Thousand Oaks: Sage Publications. Copyright © 2003, Sage Publications, is reproduced here with permission. The extract from *The Lancet,* 368 (9545), Gilbert Burnham, Riyadh Lafta, Shannon Doocy, and Les Roberts, Mortality after the 2003 invasion of Iraq: A cross-sectional cluster sample survey, pp. 1421–1428, Copyright © 2006, is reproduced here with permission from Elsevier. The extract from Civaner MM, Vatansever K, Pala K, Ethical problems in an era where disasters have become a part of daily life: A qualitative study of healthcare workers in Turkey. *PLoS ONE* 12(3): e0174162. Copyright © The Authors, 2017, is reproduced here with permission. The extract from Wetterhall, SF. And Noji, EK., Surveillance and Epidemiology. In: Eric K. Nojji, *The Public Health Consequences of Disasters,* p. 57, Copyright © 2017, Oxford University Press is reproduced here with permission.

References

Burnham, G., Lafta, R., Doocy, S., and Roberts, S. (2006). Mortality After the 2003 Invasion of Iraq: A Cross-Sectional Cluster Sample Survey. *The Lancet.* **368** (Oct. 21), p. 1422.

Civaner, M.M., Vatansever, K., and Pala, K. (2017). Ethical Problems in an Era Where Disasters Have Become a Part of Daily Life: A Qualitative Study of Healthcare Workers in Turkey. *PLoS One.* **12** (3), p. e0174162.

Kemper, E., Stringfield, S., and Teddlie, C. (2003). Mixed methods sampling strategies in social research. In: Tashakkori, A. and Teddlie, C., eds., *Handbook of Mixed Methods in Social and Behavioral Research,* 1st ed. Thousand Oaks, CA: Sage Publications, pp. 279–280.

Milken Institute School of Public Health Final Project Report. (2018). The George Washington University, Ascertainment of the Estimated Excess Mortality From Hurricane Maria in Puerto Rico, Final Project Report, August.

Patton, M.Q. (1990). Qualitative Evaluative and Research Methods (2nd ed.). Newbury Park, CA: Sage.

Pretto, E., Angus, D., Abrams, J., and **Shen, B.** et al. (1994). An Analysis of Pre-Hospital Mortality in an Earthquake. *Prehospital and Disaster Medicine*. **9** (2), pp. 107–124.

Wetterhall, S. and **Noji, E.** (1997). Surveillance and epidemiology. In **Noji, E.,** ed., *The Public Health Consequences of Disasters*. Oxford: Oxford University Press, p. 57.

Further reading

Malilay, J., Flanders, W.D., and **Brogan, D.** (1996). A Modified Cluster Sampling Method for Post-Disaster Rapid Assessment of Needs. *Bulletin of the World Health Organization*. **74** (4), pp. 399–405.

Chapter 10

Conduct a Scout Survey (Step 6)

Keypoints

We strongly recommend that a 'scout survey' of the disaster site be implemented prior to the initiation of the principal study, in order to obtain the types of detailed information required to prepare a research plan and a plan for working with a full research team during the data collection period. The scout survey step requires that one or two researchers go to the disaster site within two or three weeks following the disaster to prepare for a larger team visit, which would initiate work within two to three months post disaster. 'Scout team' visits are an essential mechanism for developing and/or revising the data collection instruments, for securing collaboration of local officials who will facilitate the study, for identifying key informants and members of the stakeholder group, and for obtaining background information needed for the sample design. We believe it is essential that the initial data collection be completed as soon as possible after the disaster event ends, in order to minimize memory loss. It is also of great importance that the primary data collection phase be conducted efficiently, within a period of approximately seven to ten days, although additional data may be added subsequent to the primary data collection period as the need for it becomes apparent. It is also likely that a data gathering effort, such as a survey involving large numbers of individuals, may continue after the main data collection team members have returned to their home institutions. The amount of thorough and detailed planning required to achieve the seven- to ten-day goal virtually mandates a pre-visit by a scout team.

Scout Team Assessment of the Disaster Zone

There are two major tasks to be accomplished during step 6. These are (1) organize and conduct a 'scout survey'; and (2) prepare a full study design and plan for working in the field during the full data collection phase (Pretto et al., 1994; Angus et al., 1997). It is advisable to allow a full week for the scout visit. We will discuss each of these tasks in turn.

The scout team process is implemented by having one or two research team members visit the disaster site, preferably within two or three weeks after the disaster, to prepare for a larger team, which would initiate work within two to three months post disaster or three to four weeks after the first interventions in disasters of long duration. The scout team visit can, of course, occur concurrent with the initiation of other steps in the eight-step model. Scout surveys are useful to inform the formation and revision of the data collection instruments, for securing collaboration of local officials and research collaborators who will facilitate the full evaluation study, and for getting a sense of the context in which the disaster occurred and within which the evaluation team will be working.

The scout visit should be organized by the evaluation team leader with the goal of accomplishing the following tasks.

◆ Convey the purpose and potential benefits of the research to political and health system leadership in the disaster area.

◆ Perform informal open-ended interviews of key officials and through this process identify and engage members of a stakeholder group.

◆ Hold the initial meeting of the stakeholder group.

◆ Visit the site of the disaster to get a clear view of the geographic context and to identify travel routes, distances, barriers, and methods by which the evaluation team will travel throughout the area.

◆ Select survey site(s) and prepare a sampling plan for both the random and purposive samples.

◆ Determine the dates for a full evaluation team visit.

◆ Select local members for the research team including the key liaison person.

◆ Collect preliminary data about damage, especially noting the geographic spread of the disaster.

◆ Make arrangement for the full evaluation team to stay for approximately seven to ten days including housing, local travel, meals, etc.

Scout Team Report

The scout team should prepare a written report which must be studied by each member of the full evaluation team. The scout team report should include a description of the disaster event, data describing the demographic and geographical context in which it occurred, major issues and barriers to the medical and public health response (preliminary assessment), unique features of the disaster, and the geographic and social/cultural context in which it occurred.

The scout team report is then distributed to each research team member at least one week prior to going to the field, allowing time for meetings to discuss the contents of the report, to address questions concerning the disaster area, and to familiarize the researchers with the unique features of the disaster including the nature of the impact, the geographic features of the impact area, and any other factors of relevance to the response.

This initial step in the preparation for the full field research effort serves multiple functions for both researchers and members of the community affected by the disaster.

- It is the ideal time for an initial meeting of the stakeholder group.
- It provides an opportunity for community leaders to assess the design of the evaluation project through their own networks, thereby building trust in the project.
- It provides time for the primary liaison person to prepare relevant members of the community for the arrival of the research team, to advise them that they will be contacted and to outline the nature of the study.
- It allows time for the team leader of the project to absorb the preliminary data that likely will have already been collected and then to organize the data collection effort.
- It provides the scout team members an opportunity to familiarize themselves with the field site and the major characteristics and issues they may encounter as the full team implements the data collection effort.
- An important result of the scout visit is that relationships are made with collaborators in the disaster area who will be essential to the conduct of the full evaluation.

Summary

It is possible to implement and complete the basic data collection phase of a disaster evaluation study within a seven- to ten-day period if the effort is thoroughly planned and the required logistics are in place. The detailed planning required to achieve such a level of efficiency is only possible if a scout team visit is carried out during which the essential ground work is prepared for a full evaluation team visit to the site of the disaster.

References

Angus, D.C., Pretto, E.A., Abrams, J., Ceciliano, N., Watoh, Y., Kirimli, B., Certug, A., Comfrot, L. et al. (1997) Epidemiological assessments of mortality, building collapse pattern and medical response after the 1992 earthquake in Turkey. Prehospital and Disaster Medicine; 12 (3): pp 222-231.

Pretto, E., Angus, D., Abrams, J., et al. (1994). An Analysis of Prehospital Mortality in an Earthquake, *Prehospital and Disaster Medicine*. **9** (2), pp. 35–45.

Further reading

The ideas presented in this chapter have their origins in **Silverman, M., Ricci, E., Gunter, M.,** and **Rawson, I.** (1980). *Field Research Methods: A Systematic Approach to the Study of Community Decision Making, Volume III.* **Health Services Research and Evaluation Unit. Graduate School of Public Health**, University of Pittsburgh, Pittsburgh, PA. Prepared for: National Center for Health Services Research, U.S. Department of Health and Human Services (IR01HSO2512).

Chapter 11

Select and Train a Field Research Team and Collect Data (Step 7)

Keypoints

Prior to beginning data collection in the disaster area, it is necessary to make extensive preparations, especially since economical use of time and resources is a prime consideration. These may be based upon the report of the scout team described in Chapter 10. The major responsibility for those preparations is assumed by one member of the evaluation team who is designated as the team leader or field research coordinator. The team leader insures the optimal use of time spent in the field and the adequate preparation of the research team and the community for the research visit. Training all members of the data collection team in the use of all data collection instruments, and in the field protocol, is an essential step in the data collection process. No matter how structured the data collection instruments may be, the reliability and validity of the data collected is a function of the ability of the data collectors to properly use the instruments. It is important to recognize that often the data required are culturally sensitive. Cultural factors are important confounders in data collection. It is essential that all data collectors are familiarized with key aspects of the culture of the area in which they will work and that persons from within the disaster region be incorporated into the research design process, the preparation of the data collection instruments, and in the data collection process itself as these individuals can assist the 'out of country' team members identify and negotiate cultural barriers and sensitivities that could impede the research. This is facilitated by conducting an initial Scout survey of the disaster zone and by using a multinational team in the design of research instruments and in the implementation of the evaluation study.

General Comments

If a scout survey has been conducted much of the background required to identify and train the data collection team will be in hand. Contacts will have been
made with potential site-specific (local) members of the research team and with
local officials who would endorse and support the evaluation effort. Also, cultural and geographic factors of importance would have surfaced.

If a pre-site visit has not been carried out (hopefully this is rare) then it is necessary to send the evaluation team leader and an assistant to the disaster site
three to five days in advance of the arrival of the full evaluation team members.
These individuals would make initial contact with relevant local officials and
the key health professionals who were responsible for the response effort and
they should be enlisted to assist with the evaluation. It would also be necessary
for this advance team to attempt to carry out, to the extent possible, the other
functions assigned to the scout team visit.

The essential criteria for the selection of the initial local collaborators is
that they:

◆ be knowledgeable concerning the disaster impact within the main
disaster area;

◆ have some legitimate leadership role in the organization and implementation of the disaster response;

◆ be knowledgeable concerning others who are involved in the disaster area;

◆ be a logical intermediary for providing liaison between the evaluation team
and the community.

For example, initial contact could be made with the community, regional,
or state emergency coordinator(s), or the chief public health official, or a
relevant governmental official. Individuals should be chosen who, due to the
nature of their position, would be able to provide liaison with other community leaders and the medical and public health personnel who could be
involved in the evaluation project. It is critical that the individual who will
serve in this liaison capacity be identified as early as possible, as he/she will
serve as the primary contact for the evaluation team while working in the
disaster area.

The timing of the field research should be negotiated with the primary liaison
person in the disaster area. When possible, a field investigation should not be
scheduled during times of additional stress or instability in the community that
may be in addition to that caused by the disaster itself. Also, the data collection
should not be scheduled when numerous participants in the program being

assessed may be absent from the community for vacations, meetings outside the community, and the like.

There are periods of time that may be more advantageous for the field research, such as when meetings are scheduled which would attract larger numbers of participants or, when special events related to the disaster evaluation may be occurring in the community which could provide an additional source of information. For example, scheduling field research in a community at a time when the leaders or major participants are convening for meetings, special training, special events, or the like, may provide evaluation team members with an opportunity to observe a number of program leaders expressing varying perspectives on the same topic or issue. This type of relatively unstructured observation(s) can provide additional information not obtained through the planned interview process.

The evaluation team leader is responsible for being knowledgeable about the political, social, and economic climate of the community, the major issues it is currently addressing, and other features that may affect conducting the research in that area. During this period, the liaison person and the team leader make their assessment of one another. It is the team leader's responsibility to clarify the research objectives and guidelines to the liaison person and to provide assurance of the confidentiality of the field research data. Building rapport with the liaison person is essential to the successful conduct of the evaluation study, since without his/her approval and support, the research may be difficult or impossible to complete.

Selecting Field Research Team Members

Several suggestions are offered for the selection of members of the data collection team:

◆ Select individuals, who have the capacity to listen, observe and keep an accurate and full record of what they see and hear.

◆ Select individuals who can follow interview schedules without 'leading' the respondent to the answer the interviewer wants or imagines is the 'truth'.

◆ The team should be multidisciplinary, ideally composed of a mix of social/behavioral scientists, public health-trained individuals, and a person with emergency/disaster medicine background.

◆ The data collection phase is quite demanding requiring long days and into the evenings for a period of up to seven to ten days. Therefore, the health and stamina of potential team members should be considered when selecting individuals for such a physically challenging effort.

Training the Members of the Data Collection Team

The quality of the data obtained during an interview is greatly dependent upon the skill of the interviewer. Therefore, the selection and training of the members of the interview team is crucial. This process is perhaps the most important aspect of data acquisition using interviews. No matter how structured and clearly worded the data collection instruments may be, the reliability and validity of the data collected are dependent upon the abilities of the data collectors to use the instruments meticulously. Time devoted to the training of these persons will be repaid in the quality of the data obtained.

As previously noted, it is important to recognize that often the questions to be asked, and the data required, are culturally sensitive. Cultural factors can become important confounders in data collection, leading to bias. It is therefore essential that all data collectors become familiar with the culture of the area in which they will be working. A reduction in culturally derived bias can be achieved by involving locals in the stakeholder group, when preparing the data collection instruments and when conducting the field research.

It is absolutely essential that prior to the start of data collection, at least one day be devoted to preparing the data collection team members for the demanding task ahead—data collection in the disaster struck region. During this training day the following should be discussed.

- Review goals and specific objectives of the evaluation project.
- Review the research plan in detail including each data collection form.
- Discuss the sampling plan.
- Review rules for the conduct of scientific interviews.
- Review behaviors expected of team members and the essential cultural aspects to be aware of when working in the disaster area

Data Collection Within the Disaster Site

Data collection in the disaster zone often involves three distinct sub-studies. It may be of value to have the evaluation team organized into three teams with each team focusing on a single sub-study.

One of the sub-studies could consist of interviews with key informants and professional participants in the disaster response, and a review of reports and other written descriptions of the disaster event, including the medical and public health response. These interviews can usually be completed during the seven- to ten-day period in which the evaluation team is in the disaster area.

A second sub-study could consist of a survey of a sample of those who live in the disaster area. This study could be initiated while the evaluation team is in the disaster zone; however, it may require a longer time period to complete, often using telephone calls or face-to-face interviews.

A third sub-study could focus on morbidity and mortality. If the 'official' (government) estimates seem credible it may only be necessary for the evaluation team to assess the extent to which a valid method was used to prepare morbidity and mortality estimates and then to be certain that the method was properly applied. In cases where the official estimates are suspect it may be necessary for the evaluation team itself to develop estimates.

The data collection process should allow for debriefing meetings each evening where team members come together discuss what was learned during the day's data collection effort. These meetings are especially important while conducting the face-to-face interviews of key informants because they allow team members to cross check information received from those interviewed each day, looking for consistencies and inconsistencies in the information obtained from each informant. These debriefings can lead to the need to cross check or triangulate information provided by adding informants or re-contacting an informant in order to resolve inconsistencies that might have surfaced during the debriefing session.

Also, during the daily debriefing meetings, barriers encountered during the implementation of the research plan should be identified. If necessary, the research plan may be adjusted, to meet and adapt to unexpected conditions which occur during the data gathering period—this is an acceptable accommodation when doing field studies.

Ideally, in any disaster situation, concurrent (simultaneously with the disaster response) data collection is preferred, but this is usually impossible from a practical standpoint. It stands, however, that the smaller the time interval between the phase for which the evaluation is relevant and the implementation of the evaluation, the more accurate will be the data acquired.

When time permits, team members may arrange for personal observation. For example, they may want to observe in the hospital emergency department, or at the dispatch center. Systematic observation of persons within the system being examined can provide a source of validation of the information received from interviews, allows the researcher to observe strategies used by members of the disaster response team to carry out response activities, helps to substantiate or invalidate hypotheses derived from the interview sessions, and generates additional hypotheses that may be explored in later interviews. Also, observations of how informants relate to their colleagues, or other members of the system, can provide clues concerning the accuracy of the formal interview data that he/she has obtained, or to identify tensions that may exist in the system but are not readily apparent from the interview data. They may also provide an opportunity to verify informally some assumptions that developed from observations in the field and from the background literature.

Rules for Working in the Field

Semi-structured Interviews with Key Informants

Some interviews (usually in the purposive sample) will be open-ended, in-depth, and semi-structured. Prior to the interview, the researcher is provided with a topic outline which covers the field of information that should be gathered during the period of data collection. Topics in the outline should include major barriers to the implementation of the response effort and issue areas in preparation and response that have been identified by the team leader during the pre-site visit, leadership, and management of the response.

Specific respondents may require the addition of special topic areas to be covered during the interview in addition to (or instead of) the general topic areas. Such individuals may have played either more narrowly focused roles or more broadly focused roles in disaster preparedness and response than the other participants and, therefore, require modification in their interview questions in order to focus on their special domain of expertise and knowledge.

Generally, an hour is allowed for each interview in the purposive sample; however, this will vary considerably depending on the willingness of the informant to allot that amount of time and his/her availability during the period of field research. It also depends on the informant's interest in the subject, his/her enjoyment of the interview process, and his/her confidence in the researchers. Frequently, informants are hesitant to schedule more than a short period of time for an interview (half an hour to an hour), but become willing to continue the interview for much longer periods of time once the process is underway. Sufficient preparation by the researcher in interviewing techniques, knowledge of the content of the interview guide, and perception of the informant's comfort with the interview is necessary in order to use the time in the field to best advantage.

It is often not possible to discern the most critical interviews (in terms of relevant data) prior to the interview, because the informant's depth of information, willingness to communicate his/her knowledge of the situation, or his/her critical and evaluative powers are not generally known until the interview is being conducted. If the interview is not of sufficient length and more information is needed from the informant, a second interview may be scheduled or the interview may be continued by telephone after the team has left the field, if it is not possible to arrange for a time during the field research process.

In some cases, more than one researcher should be scheduled to interview an informant. Such an informant may be the liaison person in the disaster area, who should be interviewed by the entire team at the beginning and again at the end of the week; or it may be an informant that is known to have been controversial or to have had considerable influence in developing and managing the response. In such cases, it is the team leader who generally conducts this more complex interview, initiating questions and bringing the interview to a close when he/she feels the informant is ready to end it. Any of the participants in the interview may address questions to such informants. Such team interviews are useful sources for validating data on critical topics since each member of the team takes notes of the interview.

While research team members are introduced into the research process prior to their entry into the field during training sessions, training may also be conducted during the data collection phase by having them accompany a seasoned researcher on the initial interviews within the field site community.

Methods for Taking, Transcribing, and Coding Field Notes

Two basic methods are used to record interviews with key informants and professional providers. The interviews may be recorded with the permission of the person being interviewed; or, the interviewer may take notes during the interview. This is a matter of personal preference. In either case the information must be put into an organized form at some point following the interview.

Following the interviews, generally when the researchers have returned home from the field, notes taken during the interview, or the recordings, are organized so as to serve as the formal record of the interview. A useful format for creating such a record includes the following:

- The written interview record is preceded by brief comments by the researcher concerning the setting of the interview, basic description of the respondent and his/her role in the disaster response itself or preparation for the disaster response, and any observations concerning possible limits to the usefulness or accuracy of the respondent's comments.
- The content of the interview is recorded essentially as conducted, editing only where it is necessary to cluster observation on the same topic. The

interviewer may also note parenthetically where specific issues are also commented upon by other informants, or where inconsistencies are noted.

◆ We suggest that interview records be typed double-spaced with a two-inch margin on the right side. This margin is used by the interviewer to later code each paragraph by content, using the chapter numbers of the final report outline. Additionally, all dates should be circled, to highlight them for the historical chronology of events.

◆ These interview write-ups should be completed and provided to the team leader within two weeks following the return of the team from the disaster site. The task of coordinating, analyzing, and writing up the field notes into a case study of the community/region is the responsibility of the team leader or someone designated by the leader.

Etiquette and Protocols for Behavior While Collecting Data

Field Etiquette

Each interviewer is responsible for maintaining a list of his/her informants with the correct spelling of names, his or her official titles, and mailing address. The liaison person in the disaster area is also notified that he/she will be sent a draft copy of the case study for review and comment. As a courtesy to the liaison person, who has played a major role in making sure that the field research is accomplished, a final meeting should be arranged with all or some of the research team and the liaison. This meeting provides an opportunity to allay any of the liaison persons' anxieties about what the research team has found. Although it is not possible for the research team to provide a summary of the week's events for this person, it is an opportunity to review the project's goals, the use to which the information will be put and to remind him/her that the stakeholder group will have sufficient input in the presentation of findings and recommendations.

Protocols for Behavior while in the Field

The interview process and observation of the system is only part of the researcher's responsibilities. Even if the research team has been accepted into the community on the basis of its credentials and reputation for past research activity, it is still necessary for the team to continue to demonstrate its reliability and integrity while in the field. This process is accomplished by maintaining the strict confidentiality of each interview, being careful not to report to other informants what has been learned from previous interviews, and by maintaining a strict style of objectivity and non-evaluation of the community or the response effort.

This professional stance may be enhanced by the researcher's dress, manners, style of interaction with the informants, and appropriately restricting conversation in the field to the privacy of their quarters or equally neutral areas. Gossip, of the sort that indicates that the researchers are carrying information from one person to another in the community, or to others outside the community, can destroy the credibility of the team and the research itself. Research staff members must not discuss in public places what they have learned from any respondent, nor should they reveal to any respondent the comments of another (unless this is a carefully planned strategy to obtain a reaction or counter comment).

Summary

The data collection phase of an evaluative study of the medical and public health response to a disaster is extremely demanding. It requires (1) careful and detailed planning; (2) cultural sensitivity; (3) careful attention to the research protocol and rules for data collection; and (4) attention to etiquette and protocols for behavior relevant to the socio-cultural environment. Also required is a general level of fitness needed for the long days and continual movement throughout the disaster area.

Acknowledgment

The methods described in this chapter and in Chapter 10 were originally developed by Silverman, M., Ricci, E., Gunter, M., and Rawsan, I. (1980, 1999) to study community planning for emergency medical services. The methods were then modified by Ricci, E. and Pretto, E. (1991), Pretto, E. et al. (1994), and Angus et al. (1997) for use in disaster evaluation studies.

References

Angus, D., Pretto, E., Abrams, J.I., et al. (1997). Epidemiologic Assessment of Building Collapse Pattern, Mortality, and Medical Response After the 1992 Earthquake in Erzincan, Turkey. *Prehospital and Disaster Medicine.* **12** (3), pp. 222–231.

Pretto, E., Angus, D., Abrams, J., et al.(1994). An Analysis of Prehospital Mortality in an Earthquake. *Prehospital and Disaster Medicine,* **9** (2), pp. 107–117.

Ricci, E., Pretto, E., Safar, P., and Klain, M.,(1991). Disaster Reanimatology Potentials: A Structured Interview Study in Armenia: A method for Assessment of the Medical Response Disasters. *Prehospital and Disaster Medicine,* **6** (2): 159-166.

Silverman, M., Ricci, E., and **Gunter, M.** (1990). Strategies for Increasing The Rigor of Qualitative Methods in Health Services Research. *Evaluation Review.* **14** (1), pp. 57–74.

Silverman, M., Ricci, E., **Gunter, M.**, and **Rawson, I.** (1980). *Field Research Methods: A Systematic Approach to the Study of Community Decision Making, Volume III.* Health Services Research and Evaluation Unit. Graduate School of Public Health, University of Pittsburgh, Pittsburgh, PA. Prepared for: National Center for Health Services Research, U.S. Department of Health and Human Services (IR01HSO2512).

Chapter 12

Analyze Data and Prepare a Final Report (Step 8)

Keypoints

In this chapter we present an overall approach to data analysis and the preparation of a final report. We suggest that the final report should initially be organized to address each major research question. However, as the research plan is implemented, additional questions may emerge or, even more likely, the original questions could have become more nuanced. It is necessary to involve some or all members of the stakeholder groups in the preparation of findings and recommendations. Initially, a simple straightforward presentation of findings, promptly prepared, will best serve the cause of improving medical and public health response efforts. In this chapter we describe a process which will lead to the completion of the type of report that will be useful to stakeholders and decision-makers. It is essential that the report be generated in a timely manner in order to enable decision-makers to draw upon recent public memory to gain support for change where required. Some general comments about data analyses are offered; however, it is not our intent in this book to provide a full discussion about data analysis for mixed methods studies. It is therefore essential that a methodologist/data analyst be included within the evaluation team.

Give them the third best to go on with; the second best comes too late; the first never comes.
(Brown, 1999)

General Comments about Data Analysis in Mixed-method Studies

Michael Quinn Patton, whose wisdom and insights we have drawn upon frequently in this book, offers sound advice about analyzing and reporting evaluation data.

> Look first for the simplest presentation that will handle the facts. Evaluators may need and use sophisticated and complex statistical techniques to enhance analytic power or uncover nuances in data, but simple and straight forward statistical presentations are needed to give decision makers access to evaluation findings.
>
> (Patton, 1997)

In the discussion that follows we borrow further from Patton (1997). There are four distinct processes involved when an evaluator works with mixed-methods evaluation data. The first level is *description*, in which data are offered in response to the evaluation questions selected for the evaluation study. A second level of data presentation is the preparation of simple univariate or bivariate/ trivariate displays (male vs. female causes of death; severity of injury by age and location, etc.).

The next level would involve *interpretation* in which the evaluator, working with the stakeholder group, attempts to explain why the findings from the data came out the way they did. Can the findings be believed? Are there alternative explanations? Would more careful or thorough triangulation help to clarify? In this phase information/facts/data that are more contextual or situational come into play.

This may involve judgment based upon the underlying value set that is present and operative in the setting. These values, professional and cultural, will always slant the judgments made about processes and outcomes in a more positive or negative direction.

The final step in the analysis and report preparation phase is to prepare *a report of findings and recommendations*. The recommendations are statements about what aspects of the response should remain the same, what should change, what are important policy issues that should be addressed, and what can be done to assure resources are available to address future disasters? Detailed guidance about the structure and process to be followed in preparing the final report is offered later in this chapter. But first we provide some suggestions for the analysis and presentation of disaster evaluation data.

Specific Recommendations for Data Analysis

It is beyond the scope of this book to provide an in-depth discussion of the multitude of statistical and qualitative data analytic approaches that are available to evaluation scientists. What follows are general suggestions about how to organize disaster evaluation data and information. We believe that the data presentation required for the initial evaluation report will be based primarily upon 'descriptive statistics' (e.g. frequency counts and percentages, measures of central tendency, including mean, medium, mode, dispersion including range and quartiles, and measures of spread such as variance and standard deviation). Usually, data displays in graphic or tabular form are found to be useful. When data are presented in bivariate displays correlational techniques can be useful when a relationship is hypothesized to exist between two or more variables.

The same general principles apply to the analysis of qualitative data. Basic displays of qualitative information, grouped, categorized, and summarized will be sufficient for the initial evaluation report.

Following the guidance of Creswell and Clark (2013) we suggest the following approach to analyzing mixed-methods disaster evaluation data.

First, go to the research questions selected for your study. These questions should, at a minimum, address the items in the 'activities' and 'outcomes' components of the logic model.

Secondly, identify the data, both quantitative and qualitative, required to answer each question.

Thirdly, prepare a table for each question that contains quantitative and qualitative data where both are available, or draw on either data set when only one type is appropriate.

Fourth, when the quantitative and qualitative data converge, complement one another, or are in agreement, it is safe to report the finding(s) in the report. When the data sets are not in agreement the analyst has four options: (1) seek other data that may confirm one or the other finding; (2) gather new data from a different data source; (3) seek clarification or confirmation from the sources that produced the original data; or (4) report both findings and discuss the implications of the differences.

Displays of Data

In a mixed methods evaluation study several types of data will be collected as has been described in previous chapters. Some data will be obtained from relatively open-ended interviews, using interview guides, with persons who may be expected to have a broad and thoughtful perspective about the response effort. Other data will be more structured (often quantified) because it is obtained from administrative or medical records or highly structured interviews. Another category of data is that drawn from written public records such as official agency reports or journalistic accounts. Finally, some information may come from ob-servations by members of the evaluation team.

Therefore, the initial displays of data will be rather straightforward arrange-ments of 'descriptive' data, or qualitative summaries for the key research ques-tions. We suggest that this will usually be sufficient for the initial evaluation report. The challenge for the initial data analysis will be to prepare displays of the relevant data and then identify areas of consistency and inconsistency. Where data from different sources appear to lead to agreement about conclu-sions drawn, confidence in the conclusions is increased. When, on the other hand, data from different sources are not in agreement, the process of triangu-lation can be useful.

In this section we provide illustrations of how quantitative and qualita-tive data maybe presented using the International Classification of Diseases Codes (ICD).

In Table 12.1 we illustrate a display of data and 2018 ICD-10-CM codes obtained in response to the research question: What were the main causes and circumstances (mechanisms) of death during the period of impact? The data used for this example are fictitious in that they have not been drawn from an actual disaster situation.

An example of a table showing how mixed-methods data can be presented is displayed in Table 12.2. In this example we show how data gathered from two data sets, a structured survey of physicians who worked in the disaster zone (N = 20), and information contained in a set of in-depth interviews with five physicians who participated in the immediate response, can be combined. In this case the qualitative data (from in-depth interviews) and the quantita-tive data (structured survey) are in agreement. The qualitative data are used to deepen our understanding of the dilemma faced by physicians (and certainly by other medical providers) who lived and worked in the disaster zone.

Single Displays of Data

Table 12.2 illustrates the display of two types of data from one type of respondent (physicians in the impact zone) in a mixed-methods study. It is also necessary to display data that are likely to be collected in evaluation studies in separate tables, such as basic data about the number and types of injuries, the location of victims, number treated in field stations who were then transported to hospital, number of deaths by type of injury and cause, age of victims, and reports of the personal 'stories' of victims and those who attempted to assist them.

Table 12.1 Causes of death within 7 days following impact of earthquake of 7.4 magnitude by age, cause of death, and mechanisms (based on medical records)

Number of decedents	Cause of death (with ICD-10-CM codes)	Mechanism (with ICD-10 codes)
N = 5	Asphyxia from chest compression: pulmonary laceration (ICD 10 CM R09.01)	Buried under rubble from home collapse (ICD-10-CM 71)
N = 10	Asphyxia from chest compression: pulmonary laceration (ICD-10-CM-R09.01)	Factory building collapse (ICD-10-CM 71)
N = 8	Abdominal compression; hemoperitoneum; liver laceration (ICDM-CM 66.1)	Home collapse (ICD-10-CM 71)
N = 8	Abdominal compression; hemoperitoneum; liver laceration (ICD-10-CM S36.113A)	Office building collapse (ICD-10-CM 71)
N = 15	Abdominal compression; hemoperitoneum; liver laceration (ICD-10-CM S36.113A)	Home collapse (ICD-10-CM 71)
N = 30	Cerebral laceration and cranial fracture from crush injury to head (ICD-10-CM S07)	Steel beam collapse (ICD-10-CM W20.0)
N = 10	Cerebral laceration and cranial fracture from crush injury to head	Tree collapse (ICD-10-CM W20.0)
N = 2	Asphyxia from chest and abdominal compression	Collapse of daycare center building (ICD-10-CM 20.1)
Total N = 100		

Structure of the Final Report

The final report should include a comprehensive 'Executive summary' which contains information about:

1. Members of the stakeholder group, the funders of the study and the evaluation team.
2. The specific aims (goal and purpose) of the study including the context relative to the disaster.
3. The research design and methods.
4. Recommendations for future preparedness and response efforts

Table 12.2 Example display of mixed methods data for one question asked of physicians: what did you do during the first hour of the disaster? (not drawn from actual interviews)

Evaluation questions (physician survey)	Unstructured interview data: physician responses	Structured survey data: physician responses
	N = 5	N = 20
What did you do during the first hour of the disaster?	R1: I made certain that my family was safe and then went directly to the hospital.	◆ Went directly to hospital = 3
	R2: My wife and children could not be located; I participated in search and rescue looking for them. How could I do otherwise?	◆ Participated in S/R for family = 9
	R3: I experienced a serious dilemma. My family and neighbors were in the impact zone. I decided to stay and provide immediate assistance to victims. It would have been unthinkable to do otherwise. The S/R team did not arrive for several hours.	◆ Went to disaster impact zone field station = 5 ◆ Stayed in home neighborhood to assist victims = 3
	R4 and R5: Same as R3.	

Executive summaries which contain the amount of detail we are suggesting are typically 15–20 pages in length. It should be a stand-alone document because it is likely to be the only report that is widely read, even by key decision-makers.

Often, the executive summary is prepared prior to completion of the final report, and we strongly recommend that this be considered for several reasons. *First*, it forces the lead evaluator and stakeholders to cut through the huge amount of detailed information that can be accumulated by an evaluation team in order to focus on that which is essential to provide answers to the most central research questions. *Secondly*, a solid draft of the executive summary can be shared quickly with stakeholders and key participants in the disaster; as a result they are more likely to provide prompt feedback since the brevity of the report encourages a prompt response, thus providing observations of value as the final report is honed. *Thirdly*, the process of preparing an executive summary will take the research team quickly from data to findings and recommendations, assuming that ample time is allowed for reflection as the team moves on to prepare the more lengthy final report.

We suggest that the final report follow a standard outline for a scientific research report which typically includes:

- *Executive summary* (methods, findings and recommendations)
- *Introduction* to the project (who the sponsors/funders are, members of stakeholder group, and research goals)
- *Background to the event*
  - nature and date/time of the event
  - description of all background factors identified in the logic model
  - initial response (first one to three days)
  - description of the lived experience of those in the impact area from time of impact to about day 14.
  - any special background factors, e.g. weather conditions, communication problems, shortages supplies, materials, and personnel, etc.
- *Design of the evaluation study* including sampling plan and research questions
- *Methods of data collection* to include procedures, barriers to implementing the plan, and any factors affecting the quality of the data collection process and the data itself.
- *Findings* both quantitative and qualitative arranged under each research question.
- *Recommendations* for future disaster preparedness and response.
- *Appendices*
  - data not included in the body of the report
  - data collection forms
  - detailed chronology of events, first two weeks following the start of the disaster.

Process of Preparing the Final Report

The following steps may be followed in preparing the final report. The process we are proposing is designed to overcome the natural tendency to delay the tedious task of writing an evaluative report with all the detail required in a scientific report.

1) Team leader assign each section of the outline to a specific person and estimate the number of pages required and a date when a first draft should be completed. This should be completed during the second week following the return from the field of the evaluation team leader.

2) The data collected should be organized with each research question in simple straightforward tables (weeks 2–5 following return from the disaster site using primarily descriptive statistics).

3) The team leader or designee should prepare an executive summary as described above (completed within four months after return from the field).

4) Share the executive summary with the stakeholder group and obtain feedback (allow two weeks). It is also useful to share the manuscript in draft form with those in the disaster area who were found to be knowledgeable and insightful during the field visit. This will result in important 'fact checking' with the resultant correction of factual errors made inadvertently by the evaluation team.

5) Incorporate comments of stakeholders and reviewers from the disaster area. It may be necessary to obtain feedback by telecommunications in order to remain within the tight timeframe which we have suggested. Within four to five months following the return of the evaluation team from the disaster site an executive summary draft should be completed.

6) The writing team can return to the preparation of the full final report which should be completed within eight to ten months following return from the data collection process at the disaster site.

This is admittedly an aggressive writing schedule; however, it is our experience that long delays can easily occur in the report writing phase, thereby reducing the likelihood that the recommendations will be implemented due to the loss of focus by policymakers and politicians who must inevitably move on to the next pressing 'problem of the day'. We suggest that the following processes be agreed to by the members of the writing team:

♦ When writing it is always best to push on to the end of each section and then on to a complete draft of the entire report. Then, as time allows, return to each section and refine and edit.

♦ As soon as possible, share the draft with others to obtain feedback. This is frequently the most personally difficult step because it is a human quality to avoid embarrassment. If this fear becomes a barrier to sharing, it is suggested that the writer prepare an agreement with a trusted colleague to exchange initial drafts, no matter how crude the wording may be, without either one exercising judgment. At times, a third party who is a professional writer can be useful to assist with revising the manuscript.

It is difficult at times to work detailed material into the body of the text and still maintain continuity. Never allow this to slow down the writing because there is always the option of moving the detailed material to an appendix.

Other Comments about the Report

It is important to acknowledge that the most important goal for the evaluation team is to facilitate the reading and use of the report in future disaster preparedness and response efforts.

Therefore, throughout this manual we have suggested procedures that have the purpose of increasing both the utility and the actual use of the findings and recommendations. These are summarized here:

♦ Involve stakeholders in the design of the study as well as in the development of findings and recommendations.

♦ Be certain to prepare a balanced report which describes the strengths of the disaster preparedness and response effort as well as areas in which improvement is necessary. It cannot be overemphasized that the full identification and description of the aspects of the response that went well is as important as the identification of components that did not work as well as hoped. The single step of reporting the strengths of the response effort will add credibility to the evaluation thereby increasing the likelihood that the findings and recommendations will be taken seriously

♦ Be as efficient as possible in the preparation of the report with findings and recommendations appearing in an executive summary. Most people will only read the executive summary. The sooner it is put in final form, and in the hands of program and policy developers, the more likely the study will have an impact and lead to change.

Summary

In this chapter we have emphasized the importance of preparing the evaluation report promptly. We described a process to facilitate the rapid preparation of a report including key findings and recommendations. It is our belief that 'descriptive statistics' and qualitative data summaries and displays will be sufficient to inform the majority of evaluation questions. We have also described a process for promptly preparing an 'Executive Summary' and final report. If the suggestions contained in this chapter are followed, it is our opinion that the majority of Executive Summaries can be completed within three to five months following return from the field with the final report coming within eight to ten months.

Acknowledgment

Reproduced with permission from Brown, S., *Technical and Military Imperatives: A Radar History of World War 2*. Bristol, UK: Institute of Physics Publishing. Copyright © 1999, Institute of Physics Publishing.

References

Brown, S. (1999). *Technical and Military Imperatives: A Radar History of World War 2*. Bristol: Institute of Physics Publishing, p. 64.

Creswell, J.W. and **Plano Clark, V.L.** (2013). *Designing and Conducting Mixed Methods Research*, 2nd ed. Thousand Oaks, CA: Sage Publications.

Patton, M.Q. (1997). *Utilization Focused Evaluation*, 3rd ed. Thousand Oaks, CA: Sage Publications.

Further reading

Onwuegbuzie, A.J., and **Teddie, C.** (2003). A framework for analyzing data in mixed methods research. In: **A. Tashakkori** and **C. Teddie,** eds., *Handbook of Mixed Methods in Social and Behavioral Research*. Thousand Oaks, CA: Sage.

Quarantelli, E.J. (2001). Statistical and Conceptual Problems in the Study of Disasters. *Disaster Prevention and Management*. **10** (5), pp. 325–338.

Chapter 13

Ethical Considerations in Disaster Evaluation Studies

Keypoints

It is only within the recent past that bioethicists and legal scholars have begun to address the highly complex domain of ethical and legal issues related to the conduct of research in the context of disaster conditions. Since the year 2000, several national and international committees and organizations have developed guidelines for the ethical conduct of research under disaster conditions. These guidelines focus upon three unique characteristics of the disaster situation that researchers must consider: (1) the unique vulnerability of disaster victims; (2) the complications related to obtaining 'ethics review' during and immediately after a disaster impact; and (3) threats to research team members, victims, and rescue workers during the data collection period. Suggestions for managing these threats and their associated risks are offered in this chapter. The framework and suggestions are drawn from reviews prepared by the World Health Organization and by a team of bioethics and legal scholars who have carefully reviewed and summarized the relevant national and international guideline statements.

Background

This chapter is based upon the contents of two comprehensive reviews of the approximately 15 sets of guidelines which have been prepared by national and international groups since the year 2000. One report was prepared by a World Health Organization (WHO) team and published in 2015 as a training manual titled: *World Health Organization, Ethics in Epidemics, Emergencies and Disasters: Research, Surveillance and Patient Care*. It contains an informed and detailed review of ethical issues in epidemics, emergencies and disasters (WHO, 2015). The WHO report is impressive in many ways. Three WHO staff members collaborated with 19 university-based faculty drawn from five countries and Médicins Sans Frontières to produce an in-depth comprehensive report and training program for public health workers and researchers who must manage the many ethical issues that come into play when working in a disaster environment.

The second source consulted for this chapter is a report titled: *Research in Disaster Settings: A Systematic Qualitative Review of Ethical Guidelines* (Fleischman et al. 2014; Mezinska et al. 2016). This review was prepared by a team of medical/bioethics university based scholars drawn from five universities (Latvia, Hungary, Croatia, Poland, and Ireland).

In Chapter 2 we presented a classification that included five general types of research: (1) basic science research; (2) clinical research; (3) health services and health systems research; (4) population-based research; and (5) policy and advocacy research. We stated that disaster evaluation studies are usually considered to be a type of health systems research in that their primary purpose is to obtain information to improve the performance of the medical and public health preparedness and response to disasters; however, classification schemes are arbitrary and, therefore, can never be considered the final or ultimate classification scheme. In the case of disaster evaluations any single study could contain elements of two or more of the types listed.

The important point in this discussion is that, however one classifies the different types of research, the risks to participants vary significantly among the types. In clinical research, which ideally involves the random assignment of patients to control and experimental treatment groups, doing so without full informed consent would be considered highly unethical today. In population-based health surveys in which the goal is to precisely determine the existence of a health issue or health problem and the correlates of each, the threats to participants are still present, but they are of less direct severity. Informed consent may still be required and confidentiality must be guaranteed, but such studies are generally given an 'expedited review'.

In the case of evaluation and quality studies, under the review guidelines currently in place in the United States and in other countries, review by a Research Ethics Committee (Institutional Review Board) is usually not required (unless a randomized controlled trial is being used). However an ethics review could be requested by the members of the evaluation study team. So what can be suggested as recommended practice in disaster evaluations?

A Classification of Types of Challenges to Participants and Researchers in Disaster Evaluations

The WHO has identified eight core ethical issues or principles and has, further, defined their relevance in emergency situations. Table 13.1 is a reproduction of a display of this information that is contained in the WHO document which we have previously referenced (WHO, 2015: 34–35).

Fleischman et al. (2014) have identified four areas of potential risk to participants in disaster studies. These include (1) concern about the decisional capacity of respondents; (2) the vulnerability of research participants post disaster; (3) evaluating the risks and benefits of such participation; and (4) the ability to obtain voluntary informed consent. They go on to say:

> Whether it is recognized or not, disaster victims and their families frequently suffer from significant psychological and emotional distress and may show signs of acute anxiety, depression, post-traumatic stress and severe grief. These emotional factors, combined with the additional stresses of … dislocation, social disruption, family and financial strains, environmental worry, and ecological stress, may render some individuals unable to make informed choices.
>
> Thus, IRBs reviewing research studies involving disaster victims must determine whether, on balance, the benefits of any particular research endeavor outweigh the cumulative risks to individual participants.
>
> (Fleischman et al., 2014)

We add only that the above applies not only to victims but to the many EMS, hospital, public health, and NGO relief workers who are called upon to assist following a disaster. These workers may have been traumatized by what they have seen or been compelled to do. Therefore, responding to questions asked by an evaluation team may cause a serious level of discomfort.

Any disaster related evaluation study involves participant informed consent, vulnerability, privacy, and confidentiality issues at a minimum. So, what can be suggested with regard to ethics review?

For data collected within a time period shortly following a disaster event we suggest the following process.

- Initially the stakeholder group (which will always include the evaluation team leader) using Table 13.1 as a guide, should assess the threats to the participants who will be asked to provide information about their experience.
- The stakeholder group should also request of the Scout Team (Chapter 10) that they explore culturally relevant issues or concerns that the population

Table 13.1 Core ethical principles and issues covered by the main guidelines and examples of their application in emergencies

Ethical principle or issues	Definition	Examples in emergencies	Examples of guidelines that address the ethical principle or issue
Respect for people's autonomy	The duty to respect people's ability to make decisions on issues related to their health and their body, if they are competent to make such decisions; and the duty to protect individuals with impaired or diminished autonomy.	Obtaining informed consent from people affected by an emergency before their identifiable personal information or biological samples are collected and processed for research purposes	CIOMS, General principles Tri-Council Policy Statement, article 1.1 Belmont Report, Basic ethical principles
Informed consent	A process whereby potential research participants decide whether they want to participate in the proposed study after receiving information about it. The requirements for consent considered to be valid vary by guideline and regulation. In general, they agree that decisions must be made free from coercion, by a competent person who can understand the information given and appreciate the associated risks. The information given to the participant should be in a language and format suitable to the participant's ability to comprehend it		CIOMS, General principles, guidelines 4-6 Declaration of Helsinki, privacy and confidentiality, articles 25-32 Tri-Council Policy Statement, Chapter 3, The consent process
Beneficence	The moral duty to pursue actions that promote the well-being of others and the ethical obligation to maximize benefit and to minimize harm	To benefit from and have access to a vaccine in a pandemic	CIOMS, General principles Belmont Report, Basic ethical principles

Table 13.1 Continued

Ethical principle or issues	Definition	Examples in emergencies	Examples of guidelines that address the ethical principle or issue
Non-maleficence	The moral duty not to cause harm to others through interventions	Vaccine trials should involve the fewest human subjects and the fewest tests on those subjects that will ensure scientifically valid data.	CIOMS, General principles Declaration of Helsinki, Risks, burdens and benefits (articles 16-18)
Justice	Primarily distributive justice, which requires equitable distribution of benefits and burdens, i.e. distribution such that no segment of the population is unduly burdened by the harms of research or denied the benefits of the knowledge generated from it	Collecting samples from citizens of a developing country affected by a pandemic in order to develop a vaccine rapidly and ensure that the vaccine is made fairly available locally	CIOMS, General principles, guidelines 10 and 12 Declaration of Helsinki, Risks, burdens and benefits, articles 16-18 Tri-Council Policy Statement, article 1.1 and Chapter 4, Fairness and equity in research participation
Vulnerability	A status in which some people may struggle to protect their interests or be at greater risk of being exploited. This situation is usually linked to specific physical, financial, educational or social circumstances. Groups considered as vulnerable vary by guideline, but children, mentally and/or physically disabled individuals, prisoners, refugees, terminally ill patients and women are often cited as the prime vulnerable groups	Targeting women and children for surveillance during emergencies without epidemiological or methodological justification	CIOMS, General principles, guidelines 13-16 Declaration of Helsinki, Vulnerable groups and individuals, articles 19 and 20 Common rule, subparts B, C and D Tri-Council Policy Statement, Chapter 9, Research involving the First Nations, Inuit, and Métis peoples of Canada

(continued)

Table 13.1 Continued

Ethical principle or issues	Definition	Examples in emergencies	Examples of guidelines that address the ethical principle or issue
Privacy	The right of expectation not to be interfered with or to be free from surveillance or, more generally, a moral right to be left alone. In practical terms, privacy is for instance concerned with the setting in which a person's health-related information is acquired	Taking precautions to interview victims of an emergency in private places (i.e. where those not related to the study cannot see or hear them)	Tri-Council Policy Statement, Chapter 5, Privacy and confidentiality Declaration of Helsinki, Privacy and confidentiality, article 24
Confidentiality	The principle that ensures that identifiable information is kept out of reach of others. All identifiable information about individuals, whether recorded (written, computerized, visual, audio) or simply held in the memory of health professionals, is subject to the duty of confidentiality	Ensuring that identifiable data from surveillance activities are secured and not accessible by irrelevant persons (e.g. locked in filing cabinets or in encrypted files)	CIOMS, Guideline 18, Safeguarding confidentiality Tri-Council Policy Statement, Chapter 5, Privacy and confidentiality

in the disaster area may find threatening and use this information to adjust data collection instruments and processes.

◆ The stakeholder group and the evaluation team leader should identify local research ethics committees, if any exist in the disaster zone, and seek their guidance. If more exist in the disaster area then a research ethics committee closest to the disaster zone should be contacted for guidance.

◆ The evaluation team leader must assure that procedures are in place to safeguard the confidentiality of the data including that obtained from medical and administrative records.

For data to be collected concurrently, it will usually be difficult to obtain ethics committee consent for surveys and other data collection tasks. However, if the information is contained in an administrative or medical records data system, to be accessed by the evaluation team during a time period following the disaster event, the core issues of informed consent, vulnerability, privacy, and confidentiality can be addressed.

Box 13.1 Options for ethics committee review for disaster studies (prior to beginning)

Single review committee for all evaluation studies relative to a single evaluation (e.g. Oklahoma City bombing)	Evaluation studies reviewed by broadly based stakeholder group which includes victims and responders	Each study reviewed independently by ethics review committee selected by each investigator (e.g. World Trade Association attack
◆ Typically slower ◆ Less redundancy and respondent burden		◆ Often quicker ◆ Could result in redundant studies with high respondent burden
OR	OR	

Summary

The ethical issues related to disaster evaluation and research continue to be discussed by ethicists and researchers and processes for dealing with them are evolving. However, the authors of this field manual strongly encourage those who are responsible for designing and conducting evaluations to address the core ethical issues to the extent possible. Evaluators have several options for obtaining input and guidance with regard to the ethical concerns which may come into play as they design and conduct disaster evaluations and then prepare and disseminate findings and recommendations.

Acknowledgment

The extract from Fleischman, A.R., Collogan, L., and Tuma, F., Ethical Issues in Disaster Research. In: Norris, F.H., Galea, S., Friedman, M.J., and Watson, P.J., Methods for Disaster Mental Health Research, Copyright © 2014, The Guilford Press is reproduced here with permission.

References

Fleischman, A.R., Collogan, L., and Tuma, F. (2014). Ethical issues in disaster research. In: Norris, F.H., Galea, S., Friedman, M.J., and Watson, P.J., eds., *Methods for Disaster Mental Health Research*, 1st ed. New York: The Guilford Press.

Mezinska, S., Kakuk, P., Mijaljica, G., et al. (2016). Research in Disaster Settings: A Systematic Qualitative Review of Ethical Guidelines. *BioMed Control Medical Ethics.* **17**(62).

WHO. (2015). *Ethics in Epidemics, Emergences and Disasters: Research Surveillance and Patient Care.* Geneva: World Health Organization.

Further reading

United Nations Evaluation Group (UNEG). (2008). *UNEG Ethical Guidelines for Evaluation.* Geneva: UNEG.

Council for International Organizations of medical Sciences (CIOMS) with WHO, (2016). *International Ethical Guidelines for Health-related Research Involving Humans.* Geneva: CIOMS.

Collogan, L.K., Tuma, F., Dolan-Sewell, R., et al. (2014) Ethical Issues Pertaining to Research in the Aftermath of Disaster. *Journal of Traumatic Stress.* **17** (5), pp 363–372.

O'Mathuna, D.P. (2010). Conducting Research in the Aftermath of Disasters: Ethical Considerations *Joupp.al of Evidence Based Medicine.* **3** (2), pp. 65–75.

Chapter 14

Epilogue

Keypoints

In this, the final chapter, we return to the premise upon which this book has been written. We contend that the concepts and methods of evaluation science constitute the best framework for the conduct of rigorous and comprehensive evaluations of the medical and public health response to disasters. The framework is based upon a "program theory" as expressed in a "logic model". The implementation of our suggested "8 Step Model" requires the collection of both qualitative and quantitative information and data, i.e. a "mixed-methods" approach. Although we expect that the underlying framework for disaster evaluation described in this book will remain stable and useful for many years, the same cannot be said for the methods we have proposed for the collection of evaluation information and data.

In this chapter we suggest some of the emerging technologies, primarily cell phone based, that could lead to improvements in the timeliness and accuracy of the data collection process, with greater cost efficiency. In addition, analytic techniques such as spatial analysis, agent based modeling, network analysis and news media analysis have potential utility in future disaster evaluation studies. We have prepared this volume with the clearly stated hope that more rigorous and systematic evaluations of the medical and public health response to disasters will lead to improved preparation and response which will , in turn, result in a significant decrease in death and disability following these horrific events.

In this Field Manual we have asserted that a 'framework for scientific evaluation', as refined by evaluation scientists over the past 50–60 years is the best model for the assessment of the medical and public health response to disasters. It is superior to other approaches for the following reasons, it is:

- Based upon the involvement of key stakeholders which helps focus the evaluation and increases the likelihood that the results will be used to inform policy and preparedness as well as future response efforts.

- In evaluations in which randomized, controlled studies are not possible, such as disasters, an alternative framework based upon a program theory as expressed in a logic model is offered as a powerful alternative.

- It recognizes the value of a mixed-methods approach that maximizes the capacity to acquire and integrate both quantitative and qualitative data and, in so doing, benefit from the unique advantages provided by each type of data.

- And, finally, the scientific evaluation framework as described in this book, enables evaluation teams to obtain a comprehensive yet nuanced description and analysis of what went right (very important) as well as what did not work as well as intended during the medical and public health response to disasters.

We expect that the conceptual framework described in this book will remain stable for many years. However, the same cannot be said for the production, availability, and accessibility of data and information required for evaluation. The rapid advances being made in telecommunications technology, the on-the-scene concurrent coverage of disasters by journalists and broadcasters, and the widespread penetration of computer-mediated technologies that facilitate the immediate sharing of information to virtual communities and networks (social media) are rapidly creating new opportunities for data collection. The development of methods to access, catalogue, and analyze communications that occur during a disaster, through social media, is a rapidly emerging area of research (Imran et al., 2013; Kumar et al., 2014).

Further, in disaster-prone areas of the planet, evaluation teams trained in disaster evaluation are seeking opportunities to collect data as the disaster unfolds. We can expect an increase in these efforts as the teams become more experienced with the complex issues and barriers associated with concurrent data collection in a disaster setting.

Cell phone penetration throughout the world is expanding rapidly, making possible rapid concurrent data collection. Two avenues appear to be opening. The first would involve tapping into a social media network (e.g. Facebook) and analyzing the earliest communication from victims. The second, more systematic, would involve obtaining a sample of cell phone numbers and texting a set of questions to the cell phone users.

Burke and Albert (2014) have compiled and described an array of emerging and potentially useful methodologies that could be considered for disaster evaluation research. We believe that the methods described in their stimulating work including, 'spatial analysis', 'agent-based modeling', 'network analysis', and 'news media analysis' should be considered for use in future disaster evaluations. Each of these rapidly emerging methods can open new windows through which disasters may be observed.

We are hopeful that the relatively new field of disaster evaluation will flourish in the coming years, thereby leading to substantial reductions in the high levels of death and disability which continues to result from both natural and human caused disasters.

References

Burke, J. and Albert, S., eds. (2014). *Methods for Community Public Health Research*. New York, NY: Springer, Chapters 2, 3, 4, and 9.

Imran, M., Elbassuoni, S.M., Castillo, C., et al. (2013). Extracting information nuggets from disaster-related messages in social media. *Proceedings of ISCRAM*.

Kumar, S., Hu, X., and Liu, H. (2014). A behavior analytics approach to identifying tweets from crisis regions. In *Proceedings of the 25th ACM Conference on Hypertext and Social Media* (edition). Ferres, Ll and Rossi, G. eds. City: ACM. pp. 255–260.

Evaluation Questions, Indicators, and Data Sources

We suggest that each evaluation team prepare a catalogue such as the following after the evaluation questions have been identified.
Illustrative only: not intended to be comprehensive.

Before-event Phase

Questions	Indicators	Methods for data collection
1. Has the community completed a hazards risk assessment?	Existence of written risk assessment by expected entities	Survey
2. Has the community assessed vulnerability and capacity?	Existence of written assessments	Survey
3. A) Has the community prepared a disaster plan? B) Was the Health System integrated into the emergency plans?	Existence of written plan	Compliance survey
4. Has the community conducted a disaster drill (or simulation)?	Report of drill (date, time, frequency)	Compliance survey
5. How effective was inter-sectoral communication and control during the drill?	Identification of an incident commander during the drill	After action report, expert interviews

Questions	Indicators	Methods for data collection
6. Has the community revised the disaster (emergency) plan based on the drill or changing conditions in the community?		Compliance survey
7. A) Have needed personnel been trained to respond to the disaster (e.g. first responders, SAR, hospital, security, public health)? B) Was it appropriate to the hazard-risks of the community?	Evidence of training (types of training, date, time, frequency, number, types of trainees)	Compliance survey
8. Is the community prepared for a disaster?	Multiple indicators of preparedness	Compilation of tools as above

During Event Phase

Questions	Indicators	Methods for data collection
1. Was the emergency warning system activated?	Early warning systems in place Case index identification through disease surveillance	Interviews/survey of responders, community, reports
2. A) Was the needs identification carried out? B) Was the needs identification adequate? C) Was it used? If partially or no, why?	Yes/no (availability of water, food, shelter, critical healthcare services) (fully, partially, No)	Structured interview, surveys, observations Assessment checklist Survey of key participants

Questions	Indicators	Methods for data collection
3. A) Were the immediate health needs of the affected community met? B) Were there preventable morbidity and mortality? C) Were the resources and supplies context-specific?	Critical health needs met, timely meeting of needs, limited wastage of resources	Interviews with survivors, medical personnel, medical records
4. How well did the EMS, SAR, and other emergency agencies respond?	Rescuing trapped survivors Triage Stabilized and transportation of injured to health facilities Was there adequate documentation/tagging of the patients being transported?	Interviews with survivors, medical personnel Medical records
5. How did the community members respond to the disaster/emergency?	Helping critical and injured patients Supporting the responders in identifying and transport of injured and critical survivors	Interviews with survivors, community members, medical personnel
6. How well did the health facilities respond to the disaster?	Screening of patients, activation of emergency protocols in hospitals Increase capacity to respond (if no why?) Sufficient/adequate supplies and resources, labs	Interviews with survivors, medical personnel Medical records

Questions	Indicators	Methods for data collection
	Referral systems for ancillary needs in place Surveillance System in place for the emergency Documentation of the pre-hospital protocols, patients, resources Adequate and timely provision of human and material resources from other unaffected health facilities	
7. A) How well was inter-agency communications, control, and management carried out? B) Was the Health System an active part of the overall emergency/ disaster management response? C) Was there adequate documentation of process of the response?	Incident command system in place Nature of communication between agencies External and internal communication systems in place	Survey/interview of key participants
8. Was information provided to the government officials, community, and media by the nodal health facilities?	Time, accuracy, frequency, completeness	Survey/ interview of key participants, Media reports
9. How were the needs of the responders met?	Security, protective safety gear, psychological support	Survey

Questions	Indicators	Methods for data collection
10. How was safety of the affected population secured?		Survey
11. Were the psychological needs of the survivors met?		Survey
12. Were the other critical societal/community needs met?	Food, water, sanitation, shelter needs	Survey

After Disaster Phase

Questions	Indicators	Methods for data collection
1. Were people with special health needs responded to adequately?	Catering to needs of elderly, people with special medical needs (diabetes, blood pressure, disability, dialysis, etc.)	Survey
2. Were the other critical societal/community needs met?	Adequate food and water supply. Safe sanitation/waste management and housing needs. Adequate secondary infection control strategies	Survey
3. What type of support was provided to survivors to help rebuild their lives?	Employment opportunities	Survey

Acknowledgment

This appendix was created from the work of the Task Force on Quality Control of Disaster Management.

Appendix B

Resources for Program Evaluation Studies

Online Advice on Program Evaluation

How to Conduct Scientific Evaluations (Online Sites)

Introduction to Evaluation

http://www.socialresearchmethods.net/kb/intreval.htm
This is a comprehensive online textbook on program evaluation. Topics include general social science research methods and evaluation models and methods.

The Instructional Assessment Resources (IAR) Website

http://www.utexas.edu/academic/diia/assessment/iar/index.php
This site introduces various methodologies and best practices in assessing classroom instruction and learning, including applications to instructional technologies. This site answers whys and hows of assessment with lots of practical advice, and it includes sections on program evaluation and education research.

Online Evaluation Resource Library

http://oerl.sri.com/instruments/cd/instrCD.html
This site contains a number of professional development modules, including designing evaluation and data collection plans, and developing written questionnaires, interviews, and observation instruments. Each evaluation module provides steps and strategies, a scenario, a case study, and references.

Program Development and Evaluation

http://www.uwex.edu/ces/pdande/index.html
This site provides a variety of learning resources. Practical suggestions and examples can be found under 'quick tips' (e.g. planning evaluation, collecting information, analyzing data, communicating results, etc.).

Program Evaluation

http://www.extension.psu.edu/evalauation/category.html

Pennsylvania State University, College of Agricultural Sciences offers tools, tip sheets, examples, and resource lists. Tip sheets are organized by topics and are particularly useful.

The Evaluation Center

http://www.wmich.edu/evalctr/
The Evaluation Center (Western Michigan University) seeks to advance the theory, practice, and utilization of evaluation. The site provides extensive resources, such as checklists for evaluators, glossaries, a searchable evaluation library database, and reports.

Electronic Evaluation Handbooks

User-Friendly Handbook for Mixed Methods Evaluations

http://www.nsf.gov/pubs/1997/nsf97153/start.htm
The National Science Foundation aims to provide practical advice on evaluation methodology. Key evaluation concepts and various qualitative and quantitative methodologies are introduced.

Evaluation Handbook

http://www.ncela.gwu.edu/files/rcd/BE0220502/Evaluation_Handbook.pdf
This handbook is aimed for those who are involved in evaluation of education programs. However, it is useful as a general text in that it describes evaluation purposes, basic definitions of program evaluation, and how to plan, implement, and report a program evaluation.

Electronic Ethics and Standards

The American Evaluation Association has developed basic ethical guidelines and principles for evaluators.

Guiding Principles for Evaluators

http://www.eval.org/Publications/GuidingPrinciplesPrintable.asp

The Personnel Evaluation Standards

http://www.eval.org/EvaluationDocuments/perseval.html

The Program Evaluation Standards

http://www.eval.org/EvaluationDocuments/progeval.html

Professional Organizations for Program Evaluation

American Evaluation Association

http://www.eval.org/
Note: The AEA lists numerous local affiliate organizations around the United States.

International Organization for Cooperation in Evaluation

http://ioce.net/members/eval_associations.shtml
Note: The IOCE lists a large number of links to evaluation professional organizations around the globe.

Journals for Program Evaluation

Below are listed a variety of professional journals dedicated to program evaluation for all types of programs. The journals with asterisks (*) indicate journals are highly practice oriented.

- *American Journal of Evaluation*
- *American Educational Research Journal*
- *Assessment and Evaluation in Higher Education*
- *Canadian Journal of Program Evaluation*
- *Educational Evaluation and Policy Analysis*
- *Educational Research and Evaluation*
- *Evaluation Review*
- *Evaluation*
- **New Directions for Evaluation*
- **Practical Assessment, Research and Evaluation* (free online journal) http://pareonline.net/

Appendix C

Questionnaires Used in Past Evaluation Studies

The data collection instruments contained in Appendix C have evolved from those used by the Disaster Reanimatology Study Group of the University of Pittsburgh to investigate causes of death and injury following severe earthquakes in Armenia, Costa Rica, and Turkey. The data collection effort has expanded conceptually since those studies were conducted; therefore, the forms presented in this appendix are designed to reflect the expanded frame of reference described in this field manual. Although they are designed for earthquake-related disasters, they can serve as models for evaluation following any large disaster. Five data collection forms are offered as examples for consideration by disaster evaluation teams.

1 Victim data summary form

   This form may be used to record data drawn from medical records for a sample of victims who were injured or who died

2 Interview with residents in disaster zone

3 Interview with local disaster response coordinators/health care professionals/search and rescue personnel

4 Chronology of events; background data: major barriers and facilitators

5 Verbal autopsy

FORM 1

Victim Data Summary (Collected from Medical Records of Those Who Were Injured or Died)

F1 - 1 Source of information:

    ○ Hospital record

    ○ Autopsy record

    ○ Both

F1 - 2 Patient identification:

    ○ Name: _____

    ○ Hospital record no. _____

F1 - 3 Initial treatment:

    ○ Time: _____

    ○ Date: _____

    ○ Provided by: _____

    ○ Place treatment provided: _____

    ○ Primary: _____

    ○ Secondary: _____

    ○ Other treatment: _____

F1 - 5 Admitted to:

    ○ Ward

    ○ ICU

    ○ OR

    ○ Seen/Discharged

    ○ Morgue:

    ○ Other (Specify): _____

F1 - 6 Discharge:

    ○ Date of discharge: _____

    ○ Primary Dx: _____

    ○ Secondary Dx: _____

    ○ Tertiary Dx: _____

F1 - 7 Surgery: Was it performed?

    ○ Yes

    ○ No

Skip To: F1 - 8 If Surgery: Was it performed?!= Yes

F1 - 7a What procedure(s) were performed?

_____

_____

_____

F1 - 8 Transport: How did the patient arrive to treatment area?

   ○ Private vehicle:

   ○ Ambulance:

   ○ Helicopter:

   ○ Other (Specify): _____

F1 - 8a Explain:

_____

_____

_____

F1 - 9 Field Care: What treatments were provided to the victim before arrival to a treatment facility? [Check all that apply]

   ☐ None

   ☐ IV

   ☐ ET tube

   ☐ CT scan

   ☐ trach

   ☐ CPR

   ☐ burn care

   ☐ antibiotics

   ☐ traction

   ☐ other:

Display This Question:

If Field Care: What treatments were provided to the victim before arrival to a treatment faci... = other:

F1 - 9a Please describe:

_____

_____

_____

F1 - 10 Cause of death?:

_____

_____

_____

F1 - 11 Estimated time of death?

_____

F1 - 12 Was an autopsy performed?

○ Yes

○ No

Skip To: F1 - 13 If Was an autopsy performed? = No

F1 - 12a Final diagnoses:

○ Primary _____

○ Secondary: _____

○ Tertiary: _____

F1 - 13 PLEASE DETAIL OTHER POINTS AS APPROPRIATE:

_____

_____

_____

_____

_____

FORM 2

Interview For Residents In Earthquake Zone

INTRODUCTION: Explain purpose of interview; obtain consent.

SECTION 1: Personal Experience

F2 - 1 What is your name?

_____

F2 - 2 Site of Interview?

_____

F2 - 3 Where is your home (address)?

_____

F2 - 4 Where were you during the first few hours after the earthquake?

_____

SECTION 2: Personal Description of Experience

F2 - 5 Please describe where you were and what you did at the time the earthquake struck - take me through your personal experience (RECORD):

_____

_____

_____

_____

_____

SECTION 3: Injury

F2 - 6 Were you injured?

○ Yes

○ No

Skip To: Form 2 - Section 4 If Were you injured? = No

F2 - 7 What was your injury? [Check yes or no for each of the following:]

	Yes	No
Mild abrasion/ laceration/ contusion:	○	○
Fracture:	○	○
Head injury (e.g. concussion):	○	○
Dust inhalation	○	○
Other:	○	○

Display This Question:
What was your injury? [Check yes or no for each of the following:] = Other: [Yes]

F2 -7a If other, explain:

_____

F2 - 8 How were you injured? [Check yes or no for each of the following:]

	Yes	No
Hit by falling debris inside building	○	○
Bit by falling debris outside building	○	○
Fall (from high place)	○	○
Cut or injured while removing debris	○	○
Injured while helping others	○	○
Intentional violence	○	○
Other	○	○
Don't Know	○	○

SECTION 4: Location

F2 - 9 Were you inside or outside a building?

    ○ inside

    ○ outside

Skip To: F2 - 12 If Were you inside or outside a building? = inside

F2 - 10 [Outside:] If outside, where were you?

    ○ Urban Street

    ○ Suburban or village street

    ○ Open ground

    ○ Other (specify): _____

F2 - 11 Were you in a vehicle?

    ○ Yes (please describe): _____
    _____

    ○ No

Skip To: Form 2 - Section 5 If Were you in a vehicle? = Yes (please describe):
Skip To: Form 2 - Section 5 If Were you in a vehicle? = No

F2 - 12 [Inside:] What was the name and/or address of the building?

_____

F2 - 13 What was the building used for?

    ○ Your home

    ○ Someone else's home

    ○ School

    ○ Factory

    ○ Office building

○ Hospital

○ Church

○ Shop/store

○ Other (specify): _____

F2 - 14 What type of building were you in?

○ Shanty construction

○ Timber

○ Masonry/stone

○ Concrete block

○ Reinforced concrete

○ Don't know

F2 - 15 How many floors did it have?

_____

F2 - 16 Where were you (floor/level)?

○ Basement

○ Ground floor

○ First floor

○ Other (specify): _____

F2 - 17 Where were you (location)?

○ Room

○ Hallway

○ Stairwell

○ Other (specify): _____

F2 - 18 If in a room, where were you?

    ○ Next to an outside wall

    ○ Next to a partition wall

    ○ In the middle of the room

    ○ Don't know

F2 - 19 What did you do to save yourself?

    ○ Stood under door frame

    ○ Near window

    ○ Under furniture

    ○ Didn't move/not applicable

    ○ Left building, escaped

    ○ Too frightened to do anything

    ○ Didn't know

    ○ Other

SECTION 5: Evacuation

Definitions:Trapped: Caught within a building or structure which has suffered more than trivial damage such that normal exit from the building is impaired.

Pinned: Physically restrained by an object.

F2 – 20 If you were inside, were you trapped?

    ○ Yes

    ○ No

F2 – 21 Were you pinned?

    ○ Yes

    ○ No

F2 - 22 Who freed you? [Check all that apply]

○ I freed myself

○ My family/friends

○ Firemen/Red Cross

○ Heavy rescue teams

○ Other

Skip To: Form 2 - Section 6 If Who freed you? [Check all that apply]!= a. I freed myself

F2 - 22a If you freed yourself, how did you do it?

○ Walked/scrambled out

○ Freed myself with my own hands

○ Freed myself by use of improvised tools

F2 - 23 Can you try to estimate how long it took you to be freed?

○ 0–5 minutes

○ <1 hour

○ <8 hours

○ <24 hours

○ >24 hours

○ Don't know

SECTION 6: Rescue Response

F2 - 24 Were you physically able to help others?

○ Yes

○ No

F2 - 25 Once you were able to move around, what did you do first?

- ○ Ran to safety
- ○ Tried to help victims where you were
- ○ Looked for a local person who was taking charge
- ○ Ran in search of a formal authority
- ○ Nothing initially die to fear or confusion
- ○ Other

F2 - 26 If you tried to help others, with whom did you work? [Check all that apply]

- ☐ Alone
- ☐ Lay public
- ☐ Fire/police
- ☐ Red Cross
- ☐ Doctors/nurses
- ☐ Other

F2 - 27 How did you know where to go or look? [Check all that apply]

- ☐ Guessed
- ☐ Knew where they were before the earthquake struck
- ☐ Saw or heard people in the debris or building
- ☐ Told by people at the site
- ☐ Instructed by team leader or commander
- ☐ Used by prior knowledge and training
- ☐ Sensing equipment
- ☐ Dogs
- ☐ Other

F2 - 28 What tools if any did you use? [Check all that apply]

- ○ Bare hands
- ○ Hand tools
- ○ Improvised tools
- ○ Hand-held power tools
- ○ Heavy rescue/construction equipment
- ○ Other

F2 - 29 Where did these tools come from?

- ○ Own tools
- ○ Construction/agriculture
- ○ Fire dept
- ○ Relief agency
- ○ Other

SECTION 7: Medical/First aid training

F2 - 30 Have you had any first aid training?

- ○ Yes
- ○ No

F2 - 31 What type of first aid training did you have? [Check all that apply]

- ○ Previous basic first aid course
- ○ First responder
- ○ Paramedic
- ○ Doctor/nurse
- ○ Other

F2 - 32 Where did you receive your training?

- O Self-taught
- O Fire
- O Police
- O Army
- O Red crescent
- O Other

SECTION 8: Medical Response

F2 - 33 Did you try to treat anyone for their injuries?

- O Yes
- O No

F2 - 34 If yes, what did you do?

- O Airway management
- O Mouth to mouth ventilation
- O Hemorrhage
- O First aid
- O Cardiac massage
- O Splinting of fractures
- O Other

F2 - 35 If no, why not?

- ○ No training
- ○ Forgotten techniques
- ○ Too emotionally upset
- ○ No or inadequate supplies
- ○ No need
- ○ Thought it was better to transport rapidly to hospital
- ○ Thought it was better to leave victim in place until medical help came
- ○ Other

FORM 3

Interview With Local Disaster Response Coordinators/ Health Care Personnel/Search and Rescue Personnel

INTRODUCTION: PURPOSE OF INTERVIEW

F3 - 1 RESPONSIBILITIES What was your role in the response to this disaster?

_____

_____

_____

_____

_____

F3 – 2 How many people were living in that area or community?

○ < 100

○ 100-1000

○ >1000

○ other: _____

F3 - 3 How many were injured? [Enter #]:

_____

F3 – 4 How many died?
[Enter #]:

_____

F3 – 5 What type of medical facilities were available in your community?

	Yes	No
a. clinic	O	O
b. hospital	O	O
c. ambulance service	O	O
d. first responders (EMTs)	O	O
e. community health workers	O	O
f. other	O	O
g. don't know	O	O

F3 - 6 What response agencies were operating in your area at the time of the earthquake?

	Yes	No
a. Red Cross	O	O
b. Fire Dept.	O	O
c. Police	O	O
d. other (specify):	O	O

F3 – 7 What foreign development agencies were operating at the time of the earthquake?

O Agency A: _____

O Agency B: _____

O Agency C: _____

F3 – 8 How did these development agencies respond to the needs caused by the earthquake?

O Agency A: _____

O Agency B: _____

O Agency C: _____

F3 - 9 Here is a list of those who died and those who were seriously injured in this area.

Were there any others who should be on this list?

○ Yes

○ No

Skip To: F3 - 11 Here is a list of those who died and those who were seriously injured in this area.

F3 - 10 If yes, please list them

_____

_____

_____

_____

_____

F3 - 11 We are keen to assess what members of the lay public were able to do to help themselves or others medically (e.g. basic first aid, knowledge of splinting, head tilt, recovery or shock positioning). What, if anything, was done to help the victims before you saw them?
Answer yes or no:

	Yes	No
a. airway management	○	○
b. mouth-to-mouth	○	○
c. bag ventilation	○	○
d. hemorrhage and shock control	○	○
e. first aid/splinting fractures	○	○
f. positioning for shock	○	○
g. other:	○	○

F3 - 12 What do you think were the main causes of death?

	Yes	no
a. airway related	O	O
b. hemorrhage/shock	O	O
c. other (specify):	O	O

F3 - 13 Which medical supplies were exhausted first?

_____

F3 - 14 How long did it take for resupply?

_____

F3 - 15 Who provided them?

_____

F3 - 16 How did resupply arrive?

O Airlift

O Land

F3 - 17 Was there need for more medical, rescue, or public safety personnel in the immediate aftermath of the earthquake?

O Yes, great need

O Yes, some

O Very little

F3 - 18 What type of personnel?

	yes	no
a. Red Cross	O	O
b. Soldiers	O	O
c. EMTs	O	O
d. nurses	O	O
e. doctors	O	O
f. U.N.	O	O
g. other	O	O

F3 - 19 Were local/medical rescue personnel sufficiently prepared for this kind of event?

○ Yes

○ No

Display This Question:
If Were local/medical rescue personnel sufficiently prepared for this kind of event? = a. yes

F3 – 20 If yes, please comment:

_____

_____

_____

_____

Display This Question:
If Were local/medical rescue personnel sufficiently prepared for this kind of event? = b. no

F3 - 21 If no, please comment:

_____

_____

_____

_____

_____

F3 - 22 Do you know about any critical incident stress debriefing of victims or rescue and health workers?

○ Yes

○ No

F3 - 23 Were victims given the change to debrief with a trained mental health worker?

○ Yes

○ No

F3 - 24 Who preformed the debriefing

○ Hospital social worker

○ Red Cross

○ Government health workers

○ Private NGO

○ Other (specify): _____

F3 - 25 Please describe the psychological after-effects observed in victims.

_____

_____

_____

_____

_____

F3 - 26 Were rescue workers given the chance to debrief with a trained mental illness health worker?

○ Yes

○ No

F3 - 27 Who performed the debriefing?

○ Hospital social worker

○ Red Cross

○ Other (specify): _____

F3 - 28 Approximately how many were debriefed?

_____

F3 - 29 Please describe any problems with the debriefings:

_____

_____

_____

_____

_____

F3 - 30 Please describe any psychological after-effects you observed in rescue and health workers.

_____

_____

_____

_____

_____

F3 - 31 What symptoms and how long after the earthquake did you observe them?

	1–2 weeks	>1 month
a. anxiety	○	○
b. sleep problems	○	○
c. loss of appetite	○	○
d. marital problems	○	○
e. quit job	○	○
f. other health problems	○	○
g. other	○	○

F3 - 32 Thank you for your help in completing this questionnaire. Finally, were another earthquake to strike, what would you do differently? (with attention to timing, communication, organization, and equipment.)

_____

_____

_____

F3 - 33 Are there any other problems or issues you would like to mention?

_____

_____

_____

F3 - END OF PERSONAL INTERVIEW

FORM 4
Chronology of Events
Background Data And Major Barriers And Facilitators To The Response

Chronology of Events

It is essential to prepare a detailed list of major events from (or shortly before) the onset of the disaster event and for the 2–3 week period following the onset. The event chronology may be drawn from sources such as:

- Newspaper accounts (useful for obtaining dates/times of important events).
- Public records e.g. police, emergency response, fire department, health department, and hospital administrative reports.
- Interviews with key officials who were responsible for the response effort.

Background Data

The following topics should be covered in the evaluation report. The data for each topic can be drawn from published material showing geographic and demographic characteristics of the population, the organizations available for the disaster response, (emergency, public safety, public health, and medical personnel) and interviews with knowledgeable officials.

F4 - 1 1. General background characteristics of the region:

- ☐ populations density

- ☐ social–demographic characteristics

- ☐ geographic features/topography

- ☐ climate

- ☐ housing/construction type

- ☐ major industries

- ☐ hospitals/staffing/ beds

- ☐ ambulance services

- ☐ health/emergency personnel

F4 - 2 2. History of disaster preparedness [to include drills and evaluations of the drills (if any)]

_____

_____

_____

_____

_____

F4 - 3 3. Organizations that participated in the response

◯ Governmental _____

◯ Military _____

◯ Non-governmental _____

F4 - 4 4. Key individuals who participated in directing the response

_____

_____

_____

_____

_____

F4 - 5. How was the response organized?

during the initial onset? (1–2 days):

_____

_____

following initial onset? (3–14 days):

_____

_____

Major Barriers and Facilitators

This section should include a list of major barriers and facilitating events. What aspects of the response went as planned and what did not work as planned? The data should be drawn from interviews with key informants.

1. List of intervention activities that worked 'well' during the response:

_____

_____

_____

_____

_____

_____

2. List of issues/ barriers/ difficulties and how addressed (discuss):

_____

_____

_____

_____

_____

FORM 5

VICTIM-SPECIFIC QUESTIONNAIRE/VERBAL AUTOPSY INSTRUMENT

SECTION P (PERSONAL)

F5.P1. Do you know the name of this victim?)

Name_____

Other description if name not available).

F5.P2. Area where victim injured [if known])

F5.P3. At what point were you involved in the care of this victim?

Answer yes or no:

○ scene   _____   _____

○ local clinic   _____   _____

○ hospital   _____   _____

○ airport   _____   _____

○ other)   _____   _____   _____

SECTION L (LOCATION)

F5.L1. If involved at the scene, was the victim injured inside or outside a structure?

○ inside

○ outside

○ don't know

F5.L2. If outside, whereabouts?

○ urban street)

○ suburban or village street)

○ open field)

○ other)

F5.L3. Was the victim in a vehicle?

○ yes

○ no

F5.L4. What was the name and/or address of the building where the victim was injured?

_____

F5.L5. What was the building used for?

○ victim's home

○ someone else's home

○ school

○ factory

○ office building

○ hospital

○ church

○ shop

○ other

F5.L6. How was the building constructed?

○ shanty construction

○ timber

○ masonry/stone

○ concrete

○ don't know

F5.L7. How many floors did it have?

\#_____

F5.L8. What level was the victim at in the building?

○ ground floor

○ first floor

○ other)

F5.L9. In what section of the building was the victim located?

○ room

○ hallway

○ stairwell

○ other

○ don't know

F5.L10. If in a room, whereabouts?

○ next to an outside wall

○ next to an inside wall

○ in the middle of the room

○ don't know

F5.L11. In particular, did you know if the victim was:

○ in a door frame

○ near a window

○ under furniture)

○ other

○ don't know

SECTION S

F5.S1. On reaching this victim, was he:

○ dead

○ alive

○ don't know

F5.S2. How did you know the victim was dead?

○ obvious (cold)

○ no breathing

○ no pulse

○ other

F5.S3. How did you know the victim was alive?)

○ talking/moving

○ noticed breathing

○ felt pulse

○ other

F5.S4. Was he/she well?

○ yes

○ no

F5.S5. Did his/her eyes open?

Estimated GCS score:

○ 4 spontaneously

○ 2.5 in response to stimuli)

○ 1 none

○ don't know

F5.S6. Was the victim's speech:

○ oriented

○ confused

○ moans

F5.S7. Was the victim able to move any limb?

○ to command

○ inappropriately or to pain

○ none

○ don't know

SECTION E

F5.E1. What did you do first?

Answer yes) or no:

a. go for help   _____   _____

b. call for help)   _____   _____

c. try to help   _____   _____

F5.E2. From whom did you call or seek help?)

○ others nearby

○ Red Cross

○ police/fire

○ hospital

○ other

F5.E3. Was the victim trapped?

○ yes

○ no

F5.E4. Was the victim pinned?

○ yes

○ no

F5.E5. In the initial management of the pinned or trapped victim what was done first?

○ removal of rubble to extricate the victim

○ evaluate, protected or secure airway

○ attempt to control bleeding

○ secure IV access

○ was a tourniquet used?

○ other

SECTION MR (MEDICAL RESPONSE)

F5.MR1. Were you involved in the medical treatment of this victim?)

○ yes

○ no

F5.MR2. Did you notice any breathing problems?

    ○ yes

    ○ no

F5.MR3. What did you do for the breathing problem?

    Answer yes or no:

    a. nothing   _____ _____

    b. watched for breaths   _____ _____

    c. cleared airway   _____ _____

    d. airway from dust   _____ _____

    e. head tilt   _____ _____

    f. mouth-to-mouth   _____ _____

        or bag ventilation

    g. supplemental oxygen)   _____ _____

    h. intubation   _____ _____

    i. mechanical ventilation   _____ _____

    j. chest tube insertion   _____ _____

    k. other   _____ _____

F5.MR4. Did you notice any bleeding problems?)

    ○ yes

    ○ no

F5.MR5. What did you do for the bleeding problem?

○ nothing

○ direct pressure

○ tourniquet

○ positioning for shock

○ cardiac massage

○ pressure dressing

○ IV fluids

○ blood transfusion

○ surgery

○ other

F5.MR6. Often, in previous earthquakes, victims have been known to deteriorate on extrication. On freeing this victim, did you notice any change in their condition?

○ airway/breathing

○ cardiovascular

○ neurological

○ other

F5.MR7. If other, please explain

F5.MR8. If yes to a, b or c, in Q. MR6, please expand:

SECTION TR (TRANSPORT)

F5.TR1. In what way did you move the patient?

- ○ carried by hand
- ○ on a sheet
- ○ board or stretcher
- ○ with attention to spinal movement
- ○ with device for spinal immobilization
- ○ didn't move patient
- ○ other

F5.TR2. How was the victim transported?)

check applicable choice for each column

	(local clinic)	(hospital)	(airport)
○ private vehicle)	_____	_____	_____
○ taxi	_____	_____	_____
○ public bus	_____	_____	_____
○ animal drawn cart	_____	_____	_____
○ carried by hand)	_____	_____	_____
○ ambulance)	_____	_____	_____
○ other	_____	_____	_____

F5.TR3. SECTION T

F5.TR4. With regard to this victim, how long was it until you:

	0-10dak	<1saat	<12saat	<24saat	>24saat
a. arrived at the building	_____	_____	_____	_____	_____
b. arrived at the patient	_____	_____	_____	_____	_____
c. finally freed the patient	_____	_____	_____	_____	_____
d. airway management	_____	_____	_____	_____	_____
e. shock control	_____	_____	_____	_____	_____
f. handed victim over	_____	_____	_____	_____	_____

Index

For the benefit of digital users, indexed terms that span two pages (e.g., 52–53) may, on occasion, appear on only one of those pages.